To Rochelle,
with respect and
admiration.

Zan
December 00

OPTIMIZING THERAPEUTIC DEVELOPMENT IN DIABETES

To the millions of children and adults who battle with diabetes every moment of the day, and to the many thousands of health professionals, investigators, and pharmaceutical developers who have joined the patients to defeat this disease.

OPTIMIZING THERAPEUTIC DEVELOPMENT IN DIABETES

G. Alexander Fleming[1]
Stanford S. Jhee[2]
Robert F. Coniff[3]
Henry J. Riordan[4]
Michael F. Murphy[3]
Neil M. Kurtz[3]
and
Neal R. Cutler[2]

[1]*Worldwide Clinical Trials, Washington, D.C., USA*
[2]*California Clinical Trials, Beverly Hills, CA, USA*
[3]*Worldwide Clinical Trials, Atlanta, GA, USA*
[4]*Worldwide Clinical Trials, Philadelphia, PA, USA*

FOREWORD

A n explosion in interest in diabetes mellitus and its treatment has occurred over the last two decades. As the economic and social costs of diabetes continue to rise due to an increasing prevalence of diabetes both in the U.S. and throughout the world, the imperative to identify successful approaches to therapy increases as well. This book provides a rationale for drug discovery and development efforts directed at diabetes and its complications.

Diabetes mellitus accounts for approximately 15% of health care dollars spent in the U.S. and approximately 25% of Medicare dollars. Diabetes mellitus is the leading single cause of adult-onset blindness and end-stage renal disease. Diabetes also increases the risk of coronary heart disease and stroke, and these complications represent the major causes of the increased morbidity and mortality associated with diabetes. Nearly 60% of dollars spent for the care of diabetes in 1997 were directed at costs arising from hospitalization for the care of diabetic complications. Thus, with the aging of the U.S. population, the increased risk of developing diabetes in the older population, the increasing corpulence of the U.S. population and its impact on the development of diabetes, and a worldwide epidemic of diabetes in countries moving from poverty to prosperity, there is a clear mandate to improve the care of patients with diabetes. New therapies should be efficacious, safe, and affordable. With "evidence-based" medicine forming the underpinnings of both drug approval by regulatory agencies and payment for drug costs by insurance companies and other third-party payers, new approaches must be undertaken to identify and test new agents to treat diabetes and its complications.

This book provides an overview of diabetes mellitus in its varying forms in addition to some insights into the current understanding of the underlying pathophysiology of diabetes and its complications. Most importantly, it provides a rationale for drug development in diabetes and points out some of the pitfalls along the way to successful development strategies. The last decade has witnessed major accomplishments in developing new therapies for diabetes. However, despite the enormous success of identifying several new classes of agents to treat hyperglycemia (the biochemical manifestation of diabetes) and to treat some of the complications caused by hyperglycemia, investigators still remain remarkably ignorant both about the molecular mechanisms causing diabetes and about the mechanisms of action of some of the drugs that successfully treat it. From complexity arises opportunity. As pointed out clearly in the text that follows, type 2 diabetes mellitus, the form that affects over 90% of patients with diabetes, is a heterogeneous set of diseases with multiple genetic and environmental contributors. Yet, as scientists begin to peel away at the multiple layers of molecular defects involved in these syndromes, they reveal new targets for drug development as well. It is likely that the next decade will see new classes of compounds emerge from basic science (discovery) laboratories and work their way through clinical trials.

Clinical trials in diabetes face a number of hurdles. The recognition that type 2 diabetes usually does not respond to a single agent over a long period of time dictates that new drugs be tested in combination with existing agents. And yet, as the number of existing agents continues to increase, the demands on clinical trial design increase in parallel. Combination drug testing is important for demonstrating efficacy, but also for ruling out potentially toxic drug-drug interactions. The developing field of pharmacogenomics may help to resolve some of these problems, but its impact has not yet been felt. Underlying the problem of clinical trials for diabetes drugs is the fact that the practitioners who prescribe these drugs are becoming bewildered by the complexity of diabetes treatments and the costs associated with them. Thus, translating the findings from clinical trials into uniformly effective treatment for the majority of patients with diabetes has lagged behind the discovery and approval of the drugs themselves. Recent concerns about the potential toxicity of diabetes drugs have been highlighted in the lay press and, for some patients, have created a sense of panic. Thus, the development of drugs for diabetes is a microcosm of the entire drug development process.

The authors have "set the table" for careful consideration of what is necessary to effectively treat a disease with devastating consequences. They have highlighted the problems and the potential of identifying new agents for diabetes. They have appropriately emphasized the importance of directing discovery efforts towards agents that intercede with the microvascular and macrovascular complications of diabetes. It is likely that even before this book is printed, new drugs of different classes will enter clinical trials and will have the potential to change the outcomes of diabetes. A revolution in drug delivery technology is addressing new ways to administer insulin and novel approaches to measuring blood glucose concentrations continuously and noninvasively and yet, for the majority of patients with diabetes, relatively "simple" oral pharmacotherapy will remain the mainstay of treatment. This book should help to create a better understanding of the complexity of diabetes, the pitfalls of developing drugs for its treatment, and the need for new paradigms of clinical trial design including, but not limited to, the identification of better surrogate markers for diabetic complications.

Alan C. Moses, M.D.

March, 1999

Cambridge, MA

ABOUT THE COVER

The cover illustration, kindly provided by Dr. Peter Ulrich, represents a glycated hemoglobin molecule. The significance of this molecule to the development of therapies for diabetes is discussed in this book's Preface. Dr. Ulrich was responsible for designing the compound aminoguanidine, a promising therapy for preventing diabetic complications. Aminoguanidine inhibits the crosslinking of proteins at residues that have been glycosylated in the presence of elevated glucose concentrations.

Data for the generation of this illustration from:

Fermi G, Perutz MF, Shaanan B, Fourme R. The crystal structure of human deoxyhaemoglobin at 1.74 angstroms resolution. J Mol Biol 1984; 175: 159–174.

PREFACE

Glycated hemoglobin, the illustration on the cover of this book, is an apt metaphor for the past decade's revolution in both the understanding and therapeutics of diabetes mellitus. Knowledge about diabetes pathophysiology and clinical outcomes of intervention has exploded. In just a few years, ambivalence has given way to a galvanized commitment among informed clinicians and patients with both type 1 and 2 diabetes to seek normoglycemia and avert complications. The identification of glycated hemoglobin, specifically HbA_{1c}, as an ideal tool for monitoring chronic glycemic control was the key advance that allowed the results of the Diabetes Control and Complications Trial (DCCT) to be so compelling. The DCCT, more than any other development, settled the debate about the value of good glycemic control. The recently reported United Kingdom Prospective Diabetes Study (UKPDS) was also dependent on this monitoring tool. The UKPDS confirmed the widely held assumption that the implications of the DCCT, which included only patients with type 1 diabetes, apply to the much larger group of patients with type 2 diabetes. Both these landmark studies also clearly showed that fully safe and effective therapies do not now exist for patients with either type 1 or type 2 diabetes. That nearly 20 million North Americans are without ideal therapies for their disease has not escaped the attention of therapeutic developers.

The significance of glycated hemoglobin extends far beyond its role as a monitoring tool that has aided drug development and improved patient care. While glycation does not significantly affect the oxygen transporting function of hemoglobin, glycation of other proteins is an important factor in the pathophysiology of diabetic complications. In the presence of hyperglycemia, the non-enzymatic catalyzed linking of glucose molecules to proteins leads to a series of chemical reactions that permanently changes the glycated proteins. Ultimately, this process alters structure and impairs function of basement membranes and increases the atherogenicity of lipoproteins. In all probability, this pervasive consequence of hyperglycemia adversely affects a host of systems.

The story behind the development of HbA_{1c} as an everyday clinical test is a reminder that diabetes is not just an enormous public health problem, but is a disease that affects persons we know and love. Dr. Anthony Cerami, a biochemist whose creativity and insight extend across many therapeutic areas, was attracted to solving the problem of adequately monitoring glycemic control when his mother developed diabetes. Mrs. Cerami was, in fact, the first patient in whom HbA_{1c} was measured and the first patient whose glycemic control was managed with this test. Her first reading was above 12%, but with use of this test, her levels consistently stayed around 7%–almost normal. She lived in relatively good health for 15 years until she developed leukemia and died at age 70.

Not surprisingly, Tony Cerami's involvement with protein glycation did not stop with HbA_{1c}. He went on to discover that glycosylation of other proteins was only a first step in a sequence of chemical reactions that lead to permanent crosslinking of these molecules. He then identified aminoguanidine, the first crosslinking inhibitor to be evaluated in long-term clinical trials for treatment of a diabetic complication. Dr. Cerami, who this summer will receive the Banting Award from the American Diabetes Association, has since developed compounds that break pre-existing crosslinks. This work has enormous potential that extends beyond the treatment of diabetic complications to other degenerative processes, including aging.

From my privileged perch as an evaluator of anti-diabetes therapies at the FDA, I know that a book with the title found on the front cover is very much needed. It remains to be seen whether the pages between the covers achieve some of the aspirations for such a book. From the start, my colleagues and I acknowledged that we would be foolish to aim at a comprehensive coverage of therapeutic development for diabetes and related conditions. Instead, we have attempted to cover many of the obvious topics and have left others for another day. We also realize that much of what we present here will become dated the moment we FedEx the galley proofs to the publisher. No matter how new its cover and pages may appear, this book should be seen as a process and not as a finished product.

Sifting through the vast store of knowledge that undergirds this book leads to a feeling of utter humility. I am reminded that a person has so little to do with what she or he knows. Rather, it is largely the wisdom, example, instruction, and discoveries of others that make us who we are and determine what we know. I am filled with gratitude for the teachers in my life: my wife, my parents (both great physicians, though only my father has a medical degree), my colleagues at the NIH, FDA, and the World Heath Organization, and my colleagues in the pharmaceutical industry, academia, and most recently at Worldwide Clinical Trials, an organization with enormous talent, expertise, and achievement. I am particularly indebted to Ms. Janis Schaap at California Clinical Trials for her marvelous research and editorial work. Without her skill and gentle prodding we never would have moved beyond an aspiration and an outline. Nor can I resist the opportunity to thank my dear colleague and hero Dr. Alan Moses, Chief Medical Officer at the Joslin and professor of medicine at Harvard, for writing the foreword to this book and for years of rich collaboration, teaching, inspiration, wise counsel, and friendship. Finally, I note my deep appreciation to our patients, the reason for the efforts of the thousands of investigators referenced in this book and the most important source of learning about this disease. Patients like Mrs. Cerami are our partners in the quest to end the harm of diabetes and the only measure of our success that really matters.

Alexander Fleming

March, 1999

Washington, D.C.

ACKNOWLEDGMENT

The authors acknowledge with gratitude and admiration the exceptional scientific and editorial contributions of Ms. Janis Schaap, M.A., science writer at California Clinical Trials. Her energy and skill have been indispensable in making this book a reality.

CONTENTS

9. REGULATORY EXPECTATIONS FOR ANTIDIABETIC THERAPIES 127

10. METHODOLOGICAL CONSIDERATIONS: DIABETIC MICROVASCULAR COMPLICATIONS...........................137

1

GENERAL OVERVIEW
OF DIABETES

Diabetes mellitus is a serious endocrine disorder that is characterized by a disruption of intermediary metabolism due to insufficient insulin activity, insulin secretion, or both. It is one of the most common endocrine diseases, and is estimated to affect over 124 million individuals worldwide, 16 million of these in the U.S. alone (Amos et al., 1997; Jiwa, 1997). Moreover, the incidence of diabetes appears to be rising; recent projections based on worldwide data have predicted that the number of individuals with diabetes will reach 221 million by the year 2010 (Amos et al., 1997).

Diabetes is associated with extensive morbidity and mortality, and is currently the fourth leading cause of death in the U.S. The social and economic costs of diabetes on society are substantial. Recent estimates have placed the economic burden of diabetes in the United States at $98 billion, over half of which is attributable to premature disability and death (American Diabetes Association, 1998; Hingley, 1997). No fully effective and safe therapies for diabetes or its complications are available. Clearly, there is an urgent need to develop effective treatment approaches for this devastating disease.

The term "diabetes" is associated with a heterogeneous group of disorders, including diabetes mellitus, gestational diabetes, impaired glucose tolerance, and diabetes secondary to pancreatic disease, hormonal alterations, or genetic syndromes (Foster, 1991). Diabetes mellitus is roughly divided into two categories, type 1 or Insulin Dependent Diabetes Mellitus (IDDM) and type 2 or Non-Insulin Dependent Diabetes Mellitus (NIDDM). The elimination of IDDM and NIDDM as terms of classification has recently been recommended (Sonnenberg, 1998), based on the argument that the distinction is unclear since patients with NIDDM may also require treatment with insulin. Instead, the new classification system emphasizes the heterogeneity of type 1 and type 2 diabetes with regard to etiology and underlying pathogenic mechanisms.

TYPE 1 DIABETES MELLITUS

Definition and Diagnosis

Type 1 diabetes generally occurs in individuals under the age of 35. It has also been called "juvenile onset" diabetes due to its high incidence in children and adolescents, and is currently the most common chronic disease in this population (Skolnick, 1997). Despite its prevalence in the young, however, type 1 diabetes may in fact develop at any age (Mølbak et al., 1994). Type 1 diabetes in early childhood is distinguished by an abrupt onset of symptoms (such as thirst, excessive urination, and weight loss) and a high frequency of ketoacidosis. In addition, the presence of autoantibodies directed against insulin have been consistently reported (Mandrup-Poulsen, 1998). Older children with type 1 diabetes may exhibit high levels of autoantibodies directed against pancreatic islet cells or glutamic acid decarboxylase, while adult type 1 patients often demonstrate relatively lower levels of both islet cell and insulin autoantibodies (Mandrup-Poulsen, 1998; Karjalainen et al., 1989). Although these and other differences suggest a heterogeneity of underlying etiologies, all cases of type 1 diabetes appear to share a final pathogenic pathway. While type 1 diabetes accounts for only a small fraction of total diabetic cases, its incidence worldwide has inexplicably risen over the past few decades (Moses et al., 1995; Schoenle et al., 1994; Burden et al., 1989; Drykoningen et al., 1992). These findings have led to increased efforts to identify environmental factors which may trigger the development of type 1 diabetes, as well as strategies to prevent the disease.

Etiology and Pathogenesis

The primary pathogenic pathway for the development of type 1 diabetes is characterized by an autoimmune response which destroys insulin-producing β-cells in the pancreas. Although the mechanisms responsible for activating this autoimmune reaction are unclear,

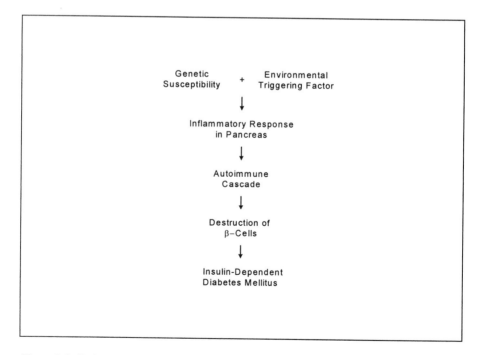

Figure 1.1 - Pathogenesis of type 1 diabetes mellitus.

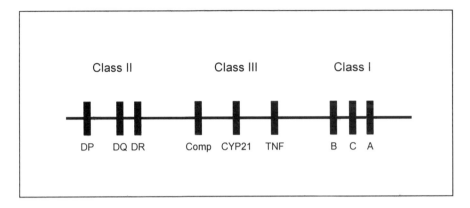

Figure 1.2 - Representation of the HLA region of chromosome 6.

both genetic and environmental factors appear to play important contributing roles. The suggested sequence of pathogenic events is depicted in Figure 1.1. According to this theory, a genetic susceptibility must first exist in order for type 1 diabetes to develop. In genetically susceptible individuals, an environmental event occurs which triggers "insulitis," or an inflammatory reaction in pancreatic β-cells. As a result of this reaction, β-cell antigens are released which contribute to a cascade of immune responses, mediated by T-helper cells, inflammatory cytokines, and macrophages. This cascade ultimately results in the selective destruction of β-cells and the appearance of diabetic symptoms.

Although efforts to identify genetic and environmental components responsible for the development of type 1 diabetes have not yielded definitive results, several factors have been implicated in susceptibility to the disease. The importance of these efforts is two-fold: determination of genetic factors may offer the best chance for identifying at-risk individuals and making accurate early diagnoses, and identification of environmental disease triggers provides good targets for prevention.

Genetic Factors

The genetic component of type 1 diabetes pathogenesis has long been recognized. Familial aggregation of type 1 diabetes has been noted in several studies (Pociot et al., 1993; Ramachandran et al., 1990), although the mechanism of inheritance remains obscure. The search for susceptibility genes is complicated by the relatively low rate of concordance between monozygotic twin pairs (approximately 50%), which suggests that non-genetic risk factors are necessary for the development of the disease (Tattersal and Pyke, 1972). Nevertheless, several candidate regions have been identified that appear to be associated with susceptibility to type 1 diabetes.

A major focus of investigation is the human leukocyte antigen (HLA) region on chromosome 6 (also called IDDM1), which encodes for gene products associated with the regulation of immune responses. It is now thought that the HLA gene region accounts for approximately 40% of the familial inheritance of the disease (Froguel, 1997; Platz et al., 1981). HLA genes can be grouped into three classes, as shown in Figure 1.2. Although early studies indicated that three HLA Class I alleles (B15, B8, and B18) were increased in diabetic patients relative to controls (Cudworth and Woodrow, 1976), characterization of the Class II genes, or HLA-D genes, has revealed an even stronger association with type 1 diabetes (Owerbach and Gabbay, 1996).

In Caucasian populations, HLA-DR3 and -DR4 alleles have consistently demonstrated a strong association with type 1 diabetes, particularly in the heterozygous DR3/DR4 combination (Field, 1989; Thomson et al., 1988; Maclaren et al., 1988). Conversely, several studies have reported that DR2 and DR5 alleles appear to have protective effects (Cavan et al., 1993; Maclaren et al., 1988; Thomson et al., 1988; Kohonen-Corish et al., 1987; Vela et al., 1987). More recently, it has been suggested that the effects of the DR3 and DR4 haplotypes are actually due to associated alleles located in the nearby DQ region. Specifically, alleles encoding for an aspartic acid at position 57 of the DQ β-chain (DQB1^{Asp57+}) are associated with resistance to type 1 diabetes, while homozygosity for DQB1^{Asp57-} appears to confer increased susceptibility (Reijonen et al., 1991; Dorman et al., 1990; Morel et al., 1988; Todd et al., 1987). In addition, individuals with alleles encoding for an arginine at position 52 in the DQ α-chain (DQA1^{Arg52+}) have also demonstrated an increased risk of the disease (Gutierrez-Lopez et al., 1992; Khalil et al., 1990). The mechanism underlying the increased susceptibility or protection conferred by these factors is unknown.

Although the HLA-D region is clearly implicated in susceptibility to type 1 diabetes, this locus cannot fully account for the familial clustering observed with this disease. Thus, the search has continued for other regions which may contribute to type 1 diabetes. For example, formal linkage analysis has revealed an association between type 1 diabetes and the human insulin gene region on chromosome 11 (also called IDDM2; Bain et al., 1992; Julier et al., 1991). Molecular heterogeneity of this region appears to be due to a variable number of tandem repeats in an area adjacent to regulatory DNA sequences that affect insulin gene expression. This suggests a possible mechanism for susceptibility to type 1 diabetes (Undlien et al., 1995; Bennett et al., 1995). The IDDM2 locus is now thought to account for approximately 10% of type 1 diabetes inheritance (Froguel, 1997).

Additionally, a candidate gene approach revealed an association of cytotoxic T lymphocyte-associated protein 4 (CTLA-4) gene polymorphism on chromosome 2 (also called IDDM12) with type 1 diabetes (Todd and Farrall, 1996). As the CTLA-4 gene encodes a receptor that mediates T-cell activation, it is a rational candidate for involvement in the autoimmune responses observed in the pathogenesis of type 1 diabetes (Nistico et al., 1996).

Environmental Trigger Factors

While formal linkage analysis has identified multiple potential susceptibility loci for type 1 diabetes, these genes do not appear to be sufficient to cause the development of the disease. As noted previously, the relatively low rate of concordance between monozygotic twins indicates a substantial environmental component in the pathogenesis of type 1 diabetes. More than 90% of type 1 cases occur in the absence of any family history (Guillausseau et al., 1997). Moreover, significant changes in the incidence of type 1 diabetes have been noted in various groups following migration to a new environment (Bodansky et al., 1992;

Siemiatycki et al., 1988). Thus, the identification of environmental "triggering" factors remains a priority of diabetes research.

Prospective studies of individuals at risk for type 1 diabetes have indicated that the onset of β-cell damage (measured by the presence of islet cell antibodies) may occur years prior to the emergence of overt symptoms (Riley et al., 1990; Tarn et al., 1988; Srikanta et al., 1983). As type 1 diabetes develops predominantly at a young age, it thus appears likely that environmental triggering factors for the disease are present as early as during gestation or shortly after birth. Recent epidemiological evidence indicates that the growing incidence of type 1 diabetes is attributable to a sharp increase in disease onset in very young children (under the age of 5), emphasizing the need to identify early environmental etiological factors (Gardner et al., 1997).

Viral Infection: Viral infections have long been suspected in the pathogenesis of type 1 diabetes. Increased levels of antibodies to the Coxsackie B enterovirus have been documented at childbirth in mothers of children who became diabetic prior to the age of 15, in comparison to mothers whose children did not become diabetic (Dahlquist et al., 1995). The presence of Coxsackie B antibodies was also found to be more prevalent in recently diagnosed type 1 diabetic patients aged 3–14 years than in a non-diabetic, age-matched sample (King et al., 1983). In addition, a recent study detected Coxsackie B virus RNA sequences in 42% of newly-diagnosed adult type 1 patients, while none were found in non-diabetic patients (Andreoletti et al., 1997). There is evidence that the Coxsackie B virus is capable of producing insulitis and β-cell destruction *in vivo* (Yoon et al., 1978; Lansdown, 1976), suggesting a mechanism for its contribution to the development of type 1 diabetes. This capacity to produce pancreatic damage may be the result of cross reactivity (molecular mimicry) between homologous sequences in the Coxsackie B virus and the β-cell autoantigen, glutamic acid decarboxylase (Vreugdenhil et al., 1998; Lonnrot et al., 1996).

A high frequency of type 1 diabetes has also been noted in young adults with congenital rubella syndrome (Menser et al., 1978; Forrest et al., 1971). This virus is associated with an increase in the concentration of islet cell antibodies, suggesting its effects are autoimmune in nature (Ginsberg-Fellner et al., 1985). The rubella virus has also demonstrated the capacity to enhance the release of cytokines such as IL-1 and IL-6 *in vitro*, which may contribute to the inflammatory response in pancreatic β-cells (Cavallo et al., 1992).

Dietary Factors: Several lines of evidence suggest that early exposure to cow's milk may contribute to the development of type 1 diabetes. For example, large, retrospective studies in multiple populations have reported that a longer duration of breast feeding is associated with a reduced risk of type 1 diabetes (Gimeno and de Souza, 1997; Virtanen et al., 1994a; Dahlquist et al., 1991; Mayer et al., 1988). In addition, disease development in animal models of type 1 diabetes can be augmented by altering the level of dietary cow's milk protein (Karges et al., 1997; Daneman et al., 1987; Scott et al., 1985). The mechanism for this effect is thought to be molecular mimicry of bovine serum albumin (BSA), a component of cow's milk, for a surface protein on pancreatic β-cells; this theory is supported by a report indicating that nearly 100% of patients with newly-diagnosed type 1 diabetes have antibodies to BSA (Karjalainen et al., 1992).

However, other evidence has revealed substantial difficulties with the "cow's milk hypothesis." For example, not all epidemiological studies have supported a link between cow's milk consumption and type 1 diabetes (Meloni et al., 1997; Bodington et al., 1994).

A recent meta-analysis of 17 case-control studies investigating the role of infant diet in type 1 diabetes found only a weak association between early exposure to cow's milk-based products and the risk of diabetes (Norris and Scott, 1996). As the majority of these studies were retrospective and based on parental memory of events that occurred years earlier, recall bias may have contributed to the lack of observed association. Additionally, recent animal studies have failed to confirm an effect of cow's milk protein on the development of diabetes (Malkani et al., 1997; Paxson et al., 1997). Moreover, the mechanism of cross-reactivity between BSA and β-cell protein has been called into question, as the finding that nearly all newly-diagnosed type 1 patients have antibodies to BSA has not been replicated (Dosch et al., 1994; Atkinson et al., 1994; Atkinson et al., 1993). Another study reported that there was no association between exposure to cow's milk and the presence of β-cell autoimmunity (Norris et al., 1996). Thus, the role of cow's milk protein in the etiology of type 1 diabetes remains controversial. A Finnish clinical study, designed to evaluate the elimination of cow's milk protein from the diets of high-risk infants, is planned (Pozzilli, 1998).

Foods rich in nitrosamines, nitrates, or nitrites have also been identified as a potential risk factor for type 1 diabetes. A prospective case-controlled study reported a significant dose-response trend for the intake of foods containing high amounts of nitrosamines and the risk of type 1 diabetes (Dahlquist et al., 1990). Prenatal exposure to nitrosamine through maternal consumption during pregnancy was also associated with the development of type 1 diabetes (Helgason and Jonasson, 1981). Nitrates and nitrites, which are partially converted into nitrosamines in the stomach, have also emerged as a risk factor for type 1 diabetes in epidemiological studies (Virtanen et al., 1994b; Dahlquist et al., 1991). Finally, a correlation was reported between the incidence of type 1 diabetes and the concentration of nitrates found in the drinking water of various communities (Kostraba et al., 1992). Experimental animal studies have indicated that prenatal exposure to nitrosamine compounds induces β-cell death, although the mechanism underlying this effect is unclear (Helgason et al., 1982).

Thus, while there are several candidate environmental triggering factors for type 1 diabetes, none appear to be necessary or sufficient to cause the disease. It is likely that a combination of factors is responsible for the pathological cascade which eventually culminates in the appearance of disease symptomatology.

TYPE 2 DIABETES MELLITUS

Definition and Diagnosis

Type 2 diabetes is the predominant form of the disease, accounting for approximately 90% of all cases. In contrast to type 1 disease, type 2 diabetes tends to emerge during middle life or later, although the incidence rate in adolescent individuals is increasing. A subtype of type 2 diabetes called maturity onset diabetes of the young (MODY) is characterized by impaired insulin secretion in young individuals who are not prone to ketoacidosis. The onset of symptoms in type 2 diabetes is more gradual than for type 1; many patients are diagnosed on the basis of elevated glucose levels (fasting glucose ≥ 126 mg/dl) rather than overt symptomatology (Foster, 1991). Alternatively, patients may go undiagnosed for several years until complications arise. Although the pathogenesis of this disease is incompletely understood, both genetic and environmental factors have been implicated.

Type 2 diabetes is characterized by relative insulin deficiency due to abnormal insulin secretion and insulin resistance in target tissues. It is unclear which of these is the root cause of the disease. Unlike type 1 diabetes, pancreatic β-cells remain anatomically intact, although they are unable to compensate for the body's reduction in sensitivity to insulin. As a result, patients with type 2 diabetes typically have normal to high absolute levels of insulin depending on the stage of the disease, but low relative insulin levels for the degree of hyperglycemia present (Foster, 1991).

Etiology and Pathogenesis

Genetic Factors

The concordance rate for type 2 diabetes in monozygotic twins is estimated at 70–80%, clearly demonstrating a strong genetic influence (Newman et al., 1987). In addition, the risk of type 2 diabetes in the offspring of two parents with the disease has been reported to be as high as 70%. Despite the compelling evidence of a genetic etiology, however, very few genetic risk factors for the disease have been identified (Davies et al., 1994). The most extensive progress in this area has been made with subtypes of type 2 diabetes which have well-defined modes of inheritance, such as MODY and maternally inherited diabetes and deafness (MIDD).

MODY is an autosomal dominant form of early-onset type 2 diabetes. It is a clinically and genetically heterogeneous disorder characterized by a primary defect in insulin secretion. Four subtypes of MODY have been identified, each associated with mutations in one of four distinct genes (Hattersley, 1998). A rare form of MODY is caused by a mutation in hepatic nuclear factor 4α, located on chromosome 20 (Yamagata et al., 1996a). A second form is linked to mutations in the glucokinase gene, located on chromosome 7 (Vionnet et al., 1992). As glucokinase acts as a glucose sensor, impairment of its activity adversely affects insulin secretion, glucose storage, and glycogen synthesis. However, this is a mild form of the disease which rarely requires medication or results in microvascular complications. A third, more severe form of MODY is caused by mutations in the gene on chromosome 12 encoding for hepatic nuclear factor 1α (Yamagata et al., 1996b). Patients with this defect are often difficult to distinguish from patients with the more common syndrome, as disease onset may occur in middle to late life. Finally, a fourth form of MODY results from a mutation of the insulin promoter factor-1 (Stoffers et al., 1997). The genes implicated in the etiology of MODY were identified with a candidate gene approach; however, this strategy has proven to be more difficult in the investigation of genes for the more common type 2 syndrome, where the mode of inheritance is less clear.

A genetic locus has also been identified for MIDD, a relatively uncommon form of type 2 diabetes that, as its name suggests, is maternally inherited and associated with the development of deafness. This disorder has been linked to a point mutation in mitochondrial DNA: a substitution of guanine for adenine at position 3243 of leucine tRNA (van den Ouwenland et al., 1992). This locus is consistent with evidence showing that type 2 diabetes follows a predominantly maternal mode of transmission, as mitochondrial DNA is inherited exclusively from the mother (Alcolado and Alcolado, 1991). Detailed evaluations of MIDD mutation carriers revealed abnormalities in insulin secretion for all subjects tested. This deficit could be due to a reduction in β-cell oxidative phosphorylation, caused by an accumulation of mutant mitochondrial DNA (Velho and Froguel, 1997). Although this mutation is well categorized in patients with MIDD, it is relatively rare among type 2 patients without hearing loss (van den Ouwenland et al., 1992).

The search for susceptibility genes associated with more common forms of type 2 diabetes has proven to be difficult. Linkage analysis is hindered by the scarcity of parents of patients with adult-onset diabetes and the limited availability of appropriate sibling pairs for evaluation (Cook et al., 1993). Furthermore, common type 2 diabetes appears to have a complex, polygenic mode of inheritance. Candidate regions under investigation include genes involved in insulin signaling or glucose metabolism, such as insulin receptor substrate 1 (Ura et al., 1996; Armstrong et al., 1996; Imai et al., 1994), glycogen synthase (Rissanen et al., 1997; Shimomura et al., 1997), the glucagon receptor (Tonolo et al., 1997; Hager et al., 1995), and Rad (ras-related protein associated with diabetes; Reynet and Kahn, 1993). At this time, however, the contributions of these genes to the pathogenesis of type 2 diabetes appear to be small and limited to particular populations of patients (Velho and Froguel, 1997).

Striking differences in the incidence of type 2 diabetes have been reported for various ethnic groups, with an increased risk for individuals of African, Asian, and Hispanic ancestry relative to Caucasians (Carter et al., 1996; Dhawan et al., 1994; Flegal et al., 1991; Harris, 1991). A higher incidence of diabetic complications and diabetes-related mortality has also been noted in these populations (Carter et al., 1996). In addition, the Pima Indians of Arizona, a genetically homogeneous group, have the highest reported prevalence of type 2 diabetes in the world, with over half of the population developing the disease after the age of 35 (Bogardus & Lillioja, 1992). However, the relative contributions of genes and environmental factors to these observed differences have not yet been elucidated. Although studies are underway to evaluate genetic differences between ethnic groups that may correlate with the incidence of type 2 diabetes, the potential influence of environmental and cultural factors cannot be disregarded.

Other Risk Factors

Insulin Resistance: Studies in numerous populations have reported that insulin resistance is a consistent risk factor for the development of type 2 diabetes (Haffner et al., 1995; Ohmura et al., 1994; Lillioja et al., 1993; Skarfors et al., 1991). Insulin resistance is also thought to be at the root of "Syndrome X," a condition manifested by hypertension, dyslipidemia, and other metabolic derangements that are associated with an increased risk of cardiovascular disease (Reaven, 1995). Insulin resistance appears to be an early development in disease pathogenesis, as reductions in insulin sensitivity have been noted up to a decade prior to the emergence of overt disease (Martin et al., 1992). It has been postulated that insulin resistance is the primary defect in type 2 diabetes, leading to β-cell exhaustion and a deficiency in insulin secretion (Bogardus, 1995; Reaven, 1995). This view is supported by evidence that severe insulin resistance due to mutations in the insulin receptor gene can result in type 2 diabetes, despite normal levels of insulin secretion (Bogardus, 1995). In addition, the degree of insulin resistance has been shown to predict the progression of glucose intolerance to type 2 diabetes in genetically susceptible individuals (Yki-Jarvinen, 1990). However, a low percentage of insulin-sensitive individuals may still develop type 2 diabetes, perhaps reflecting a heterogeneous disease pathogenesis (Haffner et al., 1997).

Obesity: Obesity is perhaps the most well-recognized risk factor for the development of type 2 diabetes. The majority of patients with type 2 diabetes are obese, and it has been suggested that obesity may be the primary contributing factor for insulin resistance in this population (Cerasi et al., 1995; Perriello et al., 1995). Physiological levels of plasma free fatty acids are elevated in obese individuals (Boden, 1997) and have been shown to inhibit insulin-stimulated glucose uptake in both healthy controls and patients with type 2 diabetes, suggesting a mechanism for the development of insulin resistance (Boden, 1998; Boden & Chen, 1995; Boden et al., 1994). Although genetics play a role in the development of obesity, environmental influences such as a high-fat diet and a sedentary lifestyle are clearly implicated; both of these factors have been identified as independent risk factors in epidemiological studies of type 2 diabetes (Gittelsohn et al., 1998; Harris, 1995; Marshall et al., 1994; Marshall et al., 1991).

Furthermore, body fat distribution is associated with the risk of type 2 diabetes. Individuals who carry their weight in the upper body (abdominal or central adiposity) are more at risk than patients who carry their weight lower, independent of the severity of obesity (Seidell et al., 1997). Abdominal adiposity may contribute to an enlargement of visceral fat deposits, which is associated with an increase in free fatty acid concentrations and alterations in endocrine function (Bjorntorp, 1996). These changes may be followed by insulin resistance and a reduction in glucose tolerance. This pathological cascade is consistent with obesity-induced insulin resistance as a primary event in the development of type 2 diabetes.

As obesity plays a significant role in the development of type 2 diabetes, a massive increase in the global prevalence of this disease has been projected based on the "Westernization" of dietary habits worldwide (O'Rahilly, 1997). Thus, the implementation of both behavioral and pharmacological strategies is an imperative response to this public health crisis.

Sedentary Lifestyle: A lack of physical activity has been shown to increase the relative risk of type 2 diabetes in multiple, diverse populations, an association that is maintained after adjustments for obesity and age (James et al., 1998; Perry et al., 1995; Manson et al., 1992; Dowse et al., 1991; Taylor et al., 1984). In one prospective study of 5990 male subjects followed for 14 years, the age-adjusted risk of type 2 diabetes was reduced by 6% for each 500 kilocalorie per week increase in energy expenditure (Helmrich et al., 1991). This protective effect was most apparent in individuals at high risk for the disease, based on obesity or a parental history of diabetes. A reduced risk of type 2 diabetes was also documented in women who engaged in vigorous exercise at least once a week in comparison to women who were less physically active, after adjustments for obesity (Manson et al., 1991).

A sedentary lifestyle may contribute to the risk of type 2 diabetes through several mechanisms. Low levels of physical activity are associated with insulin resistance, obesity, and larger amounts of visceral fat, all of which are independently associated with the development of type 2 diabetes (Samaras & Campbell, 1997). Conversely, exercise has been shown to reduce central and overall body fat (Samaras & Campbell, 1997; Buemann & Tremblay, 1996), and to enhance insulin sensitivity (Mayer-Davis et al., 1998). Even one session of exercise has been reported to enhance glucose uptake into skeletal muscle (Goodyear and Kahn, 1998). In addition, the implementation of an exercise program in sedentary type 2 patients has been shown to reduce levels of glycated hemoglobin, an indication of improved glycemic control (Schneider et al., 1984).

Low Birth Weight: An association between low birth weight and type 2 diabetes has also been noted in several studies (Lithell et al., 1996; Curhan et al., 1996; Valdez et al., 1994). Low birth weight may contribute to type 2 diabetes pathogenesis either through a reduction in β-cell mass or the early development of insulin resistance (Lithell et al., 1996; Cook et al., 1993). It is unclear, however, whether this contribution is due to fetal malnutrition or a particular genotype that predisposes individuals to both low birth weight and type 2 diabetes. This issue was recently evaluated in a study of monozygotic twins, which found that in discordant pairs, birth weights were lower for the individuals with type 2 diabetes (Poulsen et al., 1997). These results suggest that the association between low birth weight and type 2 diabetes is at least partly independent of genetics, and may be due to poor nutrition in utero.

Aging: The prevalence of type 2 diabetes increases dramatically with age (Wilson et al., 1986). Epidemiological evidence suggests that the incidence exceeds 10% in individuals over the age of 60, and ranges from 16–20 % in those over the age of 80 (Lipson, 1986). Moreover, elderly patients with type 2 diabetes are more likely to develop complications than younger patients, and demonstrate higher rates of morbidity and mortality relative to age-matched healthy cohorts (Ohno et al., 1993; Nathan et al., 1986). Prospective studies have identified age-related elevations in fasting plasma insulin (signifying increasing insulin resistance), alterations in β-cell function, and reductions in glucose tolerance, suggesting potential mechanisms for the increased incidence of type 2 diabetes in this population (Lindberg et al., 1997; Shimizu et al., 1996; Broughton et al., 1992). A deterioration of neuroendocrine function in aging may contribute to these metabolic changes (Bjorntorp, 1995). As the elderly increase both in numbers and as a percentage of the population, the incidence of type 2 diabetes is expected to grow accordingly.

CONCLUSIONS

Progress in the understanding of diabetes pathogenesis has underscored the complexity of this disease. This complexity is daunting for researchers seeking adequate therapeutic strategies; however, this complexity also represents an opportunity to identify numerous promising targets for treatment or even disease prevention. The key challenge in the successful treatment of this disease will be the translation of this basic knowledge into viable therapeutic approaches.

References

Alcolado J, Alcolado R. Importance of maternal history of non-insulin dependent diabetic patients. *BMJ* 1991; **302**: 1178–1180.

American Diabetes Association. Economic consequences of diabetes mellitus in the U.S. in 1997. *Diabetes Care* 1998; **21**(2): 269–309.

Amos AF, McCarty DJ, Zimmet P. The rising global burden of diabetes and its complications: estimates and projections to the year 2010. *Diabet Med* 1997; **14** (Suppl 5): S1–S85.

Andreoletti L, Hober D, Hober-Vandenberghe C, Belaich S, Vantyghem MC, Lefebvre J, Wattre P. Detection of coxsackie B virus RNA sequences in whole blood samples from adult patients at the onset of type I diabetes mellitus. *J Med Virol* 1997; **52**(2): 121–127.

Armstrong M, Haldane F, Taylor RW, Humphriss D, Berrish T, Stewart MW, Turnbull DM, Alberti KG, Walker M. Human insulin receptor substrate-1: variant sequences in familial non-insulin-dependent diabetes mellitus. *Diabet Med* 1996; **13**(2): 133–138.

Atkinson MA, Bowman MA, Kao K-L, Campbell L, Dush PJ, Shah SC, Simell O, Maclaren N. Lack of immune responsiveness to bovine serum albumin in insulin-dependent diabetes. *N Engl J Med* 1993; **329**: 1853–1858.

Atkinson MA, Kao KJ, Maclaren NK. Lack of immunity to bovine serum albumin in insulin-dependent diabetes mellitus. *N Engl J Med* 1994; **330**: 1617.

Bain SC, Prins JB, Hearne CM, Rodriques NR, Rowe BR, Pritchard LE, Ritchie RJ, Hall JRS, Undlien DE, Ronningen KS. Insulin gene region-encoded susceptibility to type I diabetes is not restricted to HLA-DR4 positive individuals. *Nature Genet* 1992; **2**: 212–215.

Bennett ST, Lucassen AM, Gough SC, Powell EE, Undlien DE, Pritchard LE, Merriman ME, Kawaguchi Y, Dronsfield MJ, Pociot F, et al. Susceptibility to human type I diabetes at IDDM2 is determined by tandem repeat variation at the insulin gene minisatellite locus. *Nat Genet* 1995; **9**(3): 284–292.

Bjorntorp P. Neuroendocrine aging. *J Intern Med* 1995; **238**(5): 401–404.

Bjorntorp P. The origins and consequences of obesity. Diabetes. *Ciba Found Symp* 1996; **201**: 68–80.

Bodansky HJ, Staines A, Stephenson C, Haigh D, Cartwright R. Evidence for an environmental effect in the etiology of insulin-dependent diabetes in a transmigratory population. *BMJ* 1992; **304**: 120–122.

Boden G. Free fatty acids (FFA), a link between obesity and insulin resistance. *Front Biosci* 1998; **3**: 169–175.

Boden G. Role of fatty acids in the pathogenesis of insulin resistance and NIDDM. *Diabetes* 1997; **46**(1): 3–10.

Boden G, Chen X. Effects of fat on glucose uptake and utilization in patients with non-insulin-dependent diabetes. *J Clin Invest* 1995; **96**(3): 1261–1268.

Boden G, Chen X, Ruiz J, White JV, Rossetti L. Mechanisms of fatty acid-induced inhibition of glucose uptake. *J Clin Invest* 1994; **93**(6): 2438–2446.

Bodington MJ, McNally PG, Burden AC. Cow's milk and type 1 childhood diabetes: no increase in risk. *Diabet Med* 1994; **11**(7): 663–665.

Bogardus C. Agonist: the case for insulin resistance as a necessary and sufficient cause of type II diabetes mellitus. *J Lab Clin Med* 1995; **125**(5): 556–558.

Bogardus C, Lillioja S. Pima Indians as a model to study the genetics of NIDDM. *J Cell Biochem* 1992; **48**(4): 337–343.

Broughton DL, Webster J, Taylor R. Insulin sensitivity and secretion in healthy elderly human subjects with 'abnormal' glucose tolerance. *Eur J Clin Invest* 1992; **22**(9): 582–590.

Buemann B, Tremblay A. Effects of exercise training on abdominal obesity and related metabolic complications. *Sports Med* 1996; **21**(3): 191–212.

Burden AC, Hearnshaw JR, Swift PG. Childhood diabetes mellitus: an increasing incidence. *Diabet Med* 1989; **6**(4): 334–336.

Carter JS, Pugh JA, Monterrosa A. Non-insulin-dependent diabetes mellitus in minorities in the United States. *Ann Intern Med* 1996; **125**(3): 221–232.

Cavallo MG, Baroni MG, Toto A, Gearing AJ, Forsey T, Andreani D, Thorpe R, Pozzilli P. Viral infection induces cytokine release by beta islet cells. *Immunology* 1992; **75**(4): 664–668.

Cavan DA, Jacobs KH, Penny MA, Kelly MA, Mijovic C, Jenkins D, Fletcher JA, Barnett AH. Both DQA1 and DQB1 genes are implicated in HLA-associated protection from type I (insulin-dependent) diabetes mellitus in a British Caucasian population. *Diabetologia* 1993; **36**(3): 252–257.

Cerasi E, Nesher R, Gadot M, Gross D, Kaiser N. Insulin secretion in obese and non-obese NIDDM. *Diabetes Res Clin Pract* 1995; **28**(Suppl): 27–37.

Cook JT, Page RC, O'Rahilly S, Levy J, Holman R, Barrow B, Hattersley AT, Shaw AG, Wainscoat JS, Turner RC. Availability of type II diabetic families for detection of diabetes susceptibility genes. *Diabetes* 1993; **42**(10): 1536–1543.

Cudworth AG, Woodrow JC. Genetic susceptibility in diabetes mellitus: analysis of the HLA association. *BMJ* 1976; **2**: 856.

Curhan GC, Willett WC, Rimm EB, Speigelman D, Ascherio AL, Stampfer MJ. Birth weight and adult hypertension, diabetes mellitus, and obesity in US men. *Circulation* 1996; **94**(12): 3246–3250.

Dahlquist G, Blom L, Lonnberg G. The Swedish Childhood Diabetes Study—a multivariate analysis of risk determinants for diabetes in different age groups. *Diabetologia* 1991; **34**(10): 757–762.

Dahlquist G, Blom LG, Persson LA, Sandstrom AI, Wall SG. Dietary factors and the risk of developing insulin dependent diabetes in childhood. *BMJ* 1990; **300**(6735): 1302–1306.

Dahlquist G, Ivarsson S, Lindberg B, Forsgren M. Maternal enteroviral infection during pregnancy as a risk factor for childhood IDDM: a population-based case-control study. *Diabetes* 1995; **44**: 408–413.

Daneman D, Fishman L, Clarson C, Martin JM. Dietary triggers of insulin-dependent diabetes in the BB rat. *Diabetes Res* 1987; **5**(2): 93–97.

Davies JL, Kawaguchi Y, Bennett ST, Copeman JB, Cordell HJ, Prichard LE, Reed PW,

Gough SC, Jenkins SC, Palmer SM, et al. A genome-wide search for human type 1 diabetes susceptibility genes. *Nature* 1994; **371**: 130–136.

Dhawan J, Bray CL, Warburton R, Ghambhir DS, Morris J. Insulin resistance, high prevalence of diabetes, and cardiovascular risk in immigrant Asians. Genetic or environmental effect? *Br Heart J* 1994; **72**(5): 413–421.

Dorman JS, LaPorte RE, Stone RA, Trucco M. Worldwide differences in the incidence of type I diabetes are associated with amino acid variation at position 57 of the HLA-DQ beta chain. *Proc Natl Acad Sci USA* 1990; **87**(10): 7370–7374.

Dosch H-M, Karjalainen J, VanderMuelen J. Lack of immunity to bovine serum albumin in insulin-dependent diabetes mellitus. *N Engl J Med* 1994; **330**: 1616–1617.

Dowse GK, Zimmet PZ, Gareeboo H, George K, Alberti MM, Tuomilehto J, Finch CF, Chitson P, Tulsidas H. Abdominal obesity and physical inactivity as risk factors for NIDDM and impaired glucose tolerance in Indian, Creole, and Chinese Mauritians. *Diabetes Care* 1991; **14**(4): 271–282.

Drykoningen CE, Mulder AL, Vaandrager GJ, LaPorte RE, Bruining GJ. The incidence of male childhood type I (insulin-dependent) diabetes mellitus is rising rapidly in the Netherlands. *Diabetologia* 1992; **35**(2): 139–142.

Field LL. Genes predisposing to IDDM in multiplex families. *Genet Epidemiol* 1989; **6**(1): 101–106.

Flegal KM, Ezzati TM, Harris MI, Haynes SG, Juarez RZ, Knowler WC, Perez-Stable EJ, Stern MP. Prevalence of diabetes in Mexican-Americans, Cubans, and Puerto Ricans from the Hispanic Health and Nutrition Examination Survey, 1982–1984. *Diabetes Care* 1991; **14**(7): 628–638.

Forrest JM, Menser MA, Burgess JA. High frequency of diabetes mellitus in young adults with congenital rubella. *Lancet* 1971; **2**(7720): 332–334.

Foster DW. Diabetes mellitus. In Wilson JD, Braunwald E, Isselbacher KJ, Petersdorf RG, Martin JB, Fauci AS, Root RK (eds) *Harrison's Principles of Internal Medicine, 12th edition.* New York: McGraw-Hill, 1991, pp. 1739–1758.

Froguel P. Genetics of type I insulin-dependent diabetes mellitus. *Horm Res* 1997; **48**(Suppl 4): 55–57.

Gardner SC, Bingley PJ, Sawtell PA, Weeks S, Gale EAM, The Bart's-Oxford Study Group. Rising incidence of insulin dependent diabetes in children aged under 5 years in the Oxford region: time trend analysis. *BMJ* 1997; **315**: 713–717.

Gimeno SG, de Souza JM. IDDM and mild consumption. A case-control study in Sao Paulo, Brazil. *Diabetes Care* 1997; **20**(8): 1256–1260.

Ginsberg-Fellner F, Witt ME, Fedun B, Taub F, Dobersen MJ, McEvoy RC, Cooper LZ, Notkins AL, Rubinstein P. Diabetes mellitus and autoimmunity in patients with the congenital rubella syndrome. *Rev Infect Dis* 1985; **7**(Suppl 1): 170–176.

Gittelsohn J, Wolever TM, Harris SB, Harris-Giraldo R, Hanley AJ, Zinman B. Specific patterns of food consumption and preparation are associated with diabetes and obesity in a Native Canadian community. *J Nutr* 1998; **128**(3): 541–547.

Goodyear LJ, Kahn BB. Exercise, glucose transport, and insulin sensitivity. *Annu Rev Med* 1998; **49**: 235–261.

Guillausseau P-J, Tielmans D, Virally-Monod M, Assayag M. Diabetes: from phenotypes to genotypes. *Diabet Metab* 1997; **23**: 14–21.

Gutierrez-Lopez MD, Bertera S, Chantres MT, Vavassori C, Dorman JS, Trucco M, Serrano-Rios M. Susceptibility to type I (insulin-dependent) diabetes mellitus in Spanish patients correlates quantitatively with expression of HLA-DQ alpha Arg 52 and HLA-DQ beta non-Asp 57 alleles. *Diabetologia* 1992; **35**(6): 583–588.

Haffner SM, Howard G, Mayer E, Bergman RN, Savage PJ, Rewers M, Mykkanen L, Karter AJ, Hamman R, Saad MF. Insulin sensitivity and acute insulin response in African-Americans, non-Hispanic whites, and Hispanics with NIDDM: the Insulin Resistance Atherosclerosis Study. *Diabetes* 1997; **46**(1): 63–69.

Haffner SM, Miettinen H, Gaskill SP, Stern MP. Decreased insulin secretion and increased insulin resistance are independently related to the 7-year risk of NIDDM in Mexican-Americans. *Diabetes* 1995; **44**(12): 1386–1391.

Hager J, Hansen L, Vaisse C, Vionnet N, Philippi A, Poller W, Velho G, Carcassi C, Contu L, Julier C, et al. A missense mutation in the glucagon receptor gene is associated with non-insulin-dependent diabetes mellitus. *Nat Genet* 1995; **9**(3): 299–304.

Harris MI. Epidemiological correlates of NIDDM in Hispanics, whites, and blacks in the U.S. population. *Diabetes Care* 1991; **14**(7): 639–648.

Harris MI. Epidemiological studies on the pathogenesis of non-insulin-dependent diabetes mellitus (NIDDM). *Clin Invest Med* 1995; **18**(4): 231–239.

Hattersley AT. Maturity-onset diabetes of the young: clinical heterogeneity explained by genetic heterogeneity. *Diabet Med* 1998; **15**(1): 15–24.

Helgason T, Ewen SW, Ross IS, Stowers JM. Diabetes produced in mice by smoked/cured mutton. *Lancet* 1982; **2**(8306): 1017–1022.

Helgason T, Jonasson MR. Evidence for a food additive as a cause of ketosis-prone diabetes. *Lancet* 1981; **ii**: 716–720.

Helmrich SP, Ragland DR, Leung RW, Paffenbarger RS Jr. Physical activity and reduced occurrence of non-insulin-dependent diabetes mellitus. *N Engl J Med* 1991; **325**(3): 147–152.

Hingley A. Diabetes demands a triad of treatments. *FDA Consumer Magazine*; May-June, 1997.

Imai Y, Fusco A, Suzuki Y, Lesniak MA, D'Alfonso R, Sesti G, Bertoli A, Lauro R, Accili D, Taylor SI. Variant sequences of insulin receptor substrate-1 in patients with non-insulin-dependent diabetes mellitus. *J Clin Endocrinol Metab* 1994; **79**(6): 1655–1658.

James SA, Jamjoum L, Raghunathan TE, Strogatz DS, Furth ED, Khazanie PG. Physical activity and NIDDM in African-Americans. The Pitt County Study. *Diabetes Care* 1998; **21**(4): 555–562.

Jiwa F. Diabetes in the 1990's – an overview. *Stat Bull Metrop Insur Co* 1997; **78**(1): 2–8.

Julier C, Hyer RN, Davies J, Merlin F, Soularue P, Briant L, Cathelineau G, Deschamps I, Rotter JI, Froguel P, et al. Insulin-IGF2 region on chromosome 11p encodes a gene implicated in HLA-DR4-dependent diabetes susceptibility. *Nature* 1991; **354**: 155–159.

Karges W, Hammond-McKibben D, Cheung RK, Visconti M, Shibuya N, Kemp D, Dosch HM. Immunological aspects of nutritional diabetes prevention in NOD mice: a pilot study for the cow's milk-based IDDM prevention trial. *Diabetes* 1997; **46**(4): 557–564.

Karjalainen J, Martin JM, Knip M, Ilonen J, Robinson BH, Savilahti E, Akerblom HK, Dosch HM. A bovine albumin peptide as a possible trigger of insulin-dependent diabetes mellitus. *N Engl J Med* 1992; **327**: 302–307.

Karjalainen J, Salmela P, Ilonen J, Surcel HM, Knip M. A comparison of childhood and adult type I diabetes mellitus. *N Engl J Med* 1989; **320**(14): 881–886.

Khalil I, d'Auriol L, Gobet M, Morin L, Lepage V, Deschamps I, Park MS, Degos L, Galibert F, Hors J. A combination of HLA-DQ beta Asp 57-negative and HLA-DQ alpha Arg 52 confers susceptibility to insulin-dependent diabetes mellitus. *J Clin Invest* 1990; **85**: 1315–1319.

King ML, Shaikh A, Bidwell D, Voller A, Banatvala JE. Coxsackie-B-virus-specific IgM responses in children with insulin-dependent (juvenile-onset; type I) diabetes mellitus. *Lancet* 1983; **1**(8339): 1397–1399.

Kohonen-Corish MR, Serjeantson SW, Lee HK, Zimmet P. Insulin-dependent diabetes mellitus: HLA-DR and -DQ genotyping in three ethnic groups. *Dis Markers* 1987; **5**(3): 153–164.

Kostraba JN, Gay EC, Rewers M, Hammam RF. Nitrate levels in community drinking waters and risk of IDDM. *Diabetes Care* 1992; **15**: 1505–1508.

Lansdown AB. Pathological changes in the pancreas of mice following infection with coxsackie B viruses. *Br J Exp Pathol* 1976; **57**(3): 331–338.

Lillioja S, Mott DM, Spraul M, Ferraro R, Foley JE, Ravussin E, Knowler WC, Bennett PH, Bogardus C. Insulin resistance and insulin secretory dysfunction as precursors of non-insulin-dependent diabetes mellitus. Prospective studies of Pima Indians. *N Engl J Med* 1993; **329**(27): 1988–1992.

Lindberg O, Tilvis RS, Strandberg TE. Does fasting plasma insulin increase by age in the general elderly population? *Aging (Milano)* 1997; **9**(4): 277–280.

Lipson LG. Diabetes in the elderly: diagnosis, pathogenesis, and therapy. *Am J Med* 1986; **805**(A): 10–21.

Lithell HO, McKegue PM, Berglund L, Mohasen R, Lithell UB, Leon D. Relation of size at birth to non-insulin dependent diabetes and insulin concentrations in men aged 50-60 years. *BMJ* 1996; **312**(7028): 406–410.

Lonnrot M, Hyoty H, Knip M, Roivainen M, Kulmala P, Leinikki P, Akerblom HK. Antibody cross-reactivity induced by the homologous regions in glutamic acid decarboxylase (GAD65) and 2C protein of coxsackie virus B4. Childhood Diabetes in Finland Study Group. *Clin Exp Immunol* 1996; **104**(3): 398–405.

Maclaren N, Riley W, Skordis N, Atkinson M, Spillar R, Silverstein J, Klein R, Vadheim C, Rotter J. Inherited susceptibility to insulin-dependent diabetes is associated with HLA-DR1, while DR5 is protective. *Autoimmunity* 1988; **1**(3): 197–205.

Malkani S, Nompleggi D, Hansen JW, Greiner DL, Mordes JP, Rossini AA. Dietary cow's milk protein does not alter the frequency of diabetes in the BB rat. *Diabetes* 1997; **46**(7): 1133–1140.

Mandrup-Poulsen T. Recent advances. Diabetes. *BMJ* 1998; **316**: 1221–1225.

Manson JE, Nathan DM, Krolewski AS, Stampfer MJ, Willett WC, Hennekens CH. A prospective study of exercise and incidence of diabetes among US male physicians. *JAMA* 1992; **268**(1): 63–67.

Manson JE, Rimm EB, Stampfer MJ, Colditz GA, Willett WC, Krolewski AS, Rosner B, Hennekens CH, Speizer FE. Physical activity and incidence of non-insulin-dependent diabetes mellitus in women. *Lancet* 1991; **338**(8770): 774–778.

Marshall JA, Hamman RF, Baxter J. High-fat, low-carbohydrate diet and the etiology of non-insulin-dependent diabetes mellitus: the San Luis Valley Diabetes Study. *Am J Epidemiol* 1991; **134**(6): 590–603.

Marshall JA, Hoag S, Shetterly S, Hamman RF. Dietary fat predicts conversion from impaired glucose tolerance to NIDDM. The San Luis Valley Diabetes Study. *Diabetes Care* 1994; **17**(1): 50–56.

Martin BC, Warram JH, Krolewski AS, Bergman RN, Soeldner JS, Kahn CR. Role of glucose and insulin resistance in development of type 2 diabetes mellitus: results of a 25-year follow-up study. *Lancet* 1992; **340**(8825): 925–929.

Mayer EJ, Hamman RF, Gay EC, Lezotte DC, Savitz DA, Klingensmith GJ. Reduced risk of IDDM among breast-fed children, The Colorado IDDM Registry. *Diabetes* 1988; **37**(12): 1625–1632.

Mayer-Davis EJ, D'Agostino R Jr, Karter AJ, Haffner SM, Rewers MJ, Saad M, Bergman RN. Intensity and amount of physical activity in relation to insulin sensitivity: the Insulin Resistance Atherosclerosis Study. *JAMA* 1998; **279**(9): 669–674.

Meloni T, Marinaro AM, Mannazzu MC, Ogana A, La Vecchia C, Negri E, Colombo C. IDDM and early infant feeding. Sardinian case-control study. *Diabetes Care* 1997; **20**(3): 340–342.

Menser MA, Forrest JM, Bransby RD. Rubella infection and diabetes mellitus. *Lancet* 1978; **1**(8055): 57–60.

Mølbak AG, Marner B, Borch-Johnsen K, Nerup J. Incidence of insulin-dependent diabetes mellitus in age groups over 30 years in Denmark. *Diabet Med* 1994; **11**: 650–665.

Morel PA, Dorman JS, Todd JA, McDevitt HO, Trucco M. Aspartic acid at position 57 of the HLA-DQ beta chain protects against type I diabetes: a family study. *Proc Natl Acad Sci USA* 1988; **85**(21): 8111–8115.

Moses RG, Matthews JA, Griffiths R. Dramatic increase in incidence of insulin-dependent diabetes mellitus in Western Australia [letter]. *Med J Aust* 1995; **162**(2): 111.

Nathan DM, Singer DE, Godine JE, Perlmuter LC. Non-insulin-dependent diabetes in older patients. Complications and risk factors. *Am J Med* 1986; **81**(5): 837–842.

Newman B, Selby J, King M, Slemenda C, Fabsitz R, Friedman G. Concordance for type 2 diabetes in male twins. *Diabetologia* 1987; **30**: 763–768.

Nistico L, Buzzetti R, Pritchard LE, Van der Auwera B, Giovannini C, Bosi E, Larrad MT, Rios MS, Chow CC, Cockram CS, et al. The CTLA-4 gene region of chromosome 2q33 is linked to, and associated with, type 1 diabetes. Belgian Diabetes Registry. *Hum Mol Genet* 1996; **5**(7): 1075–1080.

Norris JM, Beaty B, Klingensmith G, Yu Liping, Hoffman M, Chase HP, Erlich HA, Hamman RF, Eisenbarth GS, Rewers M. Lack of association between early exposure to cow's milk protein and beta-cell autoimmunity. Diabetes Autoimmunity Study in the Young. *JAMA* 1996; **276**(8): 609–614.

Norris JM, Scott FW. A meta-analysis of infant diet and insulin-dependent diabetes mellitus: do biases play a role? *Epidemiology* 1996; **7**(1): 87–92.

Ohmura T, Ueda K, Kiyohara Y, Kato I, Iwamoto H, Nakayama K, Nomiyama K, Ohmori S, Yoshitake T, Shinkawa A, et al. The association of the insulin resistance syndrome with impaired glucose tolerance and NIDDM in the Japanese general population: the Hisayama study. *Diabetologia* 1994; **37**(9): 897–904.

Ohno T, Kato N, Shimizu M, Ishii C, Ito Y, Tomono S, Kawazu S, Murata K. Effect of age on the development or progression of albuminuria in non-insulin-dependent diabetes mellitus (NIDDM) without hypertension. *Diabetes Res* 1993; **22**(3): 115–121.

O'Rahilly S. Science, medicine, and the future. Non-insulin-dependent diabetes mellitus: the gathering storm. *BMJ* 1997; **314**: 955–959.

Owerbach D, Gabbay KH. The search for IDDM susceptibility genes. The next generation. *Diabetes* 1996; **45**: 544–551.

Paxson JA, Weber JG, Kulczycki A Jr. Cow's milk-free diet does not prevent diabetes in NOD mice. *Diabetes* 1997; **46**(11): 1711–1717.

Perriello G, Misericordia P, Volpi E, Pampanelli S, Santeusanio F, Brunetti P, Bolli GB. Contribution of obesity to insulin resistance in noninsulin-dependent diabetes mellitus. *J*

Clin Endocrinol Metab 1995; **80**(8): 2464–2469.

Perry IJ, Wannamethee SG, Walker MK, Thomson AG, Whincup PH, Shaper AG. Prospective study of risk factors for development of non-insulin dependent diabetes in middle aged British men. *BMJ* 1995; **310**(6979): 560–564.

Platz P, Jakobsen BK, Morling N, Ryder LP, Svejgaard A, Thomsen M, Christy M, Kromann H, Benn J, Nerup J et al. HLA-D and HLA-DR antigens in genetic analysis of insulin-dependent diabetes mellitus. *Diabetologia* 1981; **21**: 1108–1115.

Pociot F, Norgaard K, Hobolth N, Andersen O, Nerup J. A nationwide population-based study of the familial aggregation of type I (insulin-dependent) diabetes mellitus in Denmark, Danish Study Group of Diabetes in Childhood. *Diabetologia* 1993; **36**(9): 870––875.

Poulsen P, Vaag AA, Kyvik KO, Moller-Jensen D, Beck-Nielsen H. Low birthweight is associated with NIDDM in discordant monozygotic and dizygotic twins. *Diabetologia* 1997; **40**(4): 439–446.

Pozzilli P. Prevention of insulin-dependent diabetes mellitus 1998. *Diabetes Metab Rev* 1998; **14**: 69–84.

Ramachandran A, Snehalatha C, Premila L, Mohan V, Viswanathan M. Familial aggregation in type I (insulin-dependent) diabetes mellitus: a study from south India. *Diabet Med* 1990; **7**(10): 876–879.

Reaven GM. Pathophysiology of insulin resistance in human disease. *Physiol Rev* 1995; **75**(3): 473–486.

Reijonen H, Ilonen J, Knip M, Akerblom HK. HLA-DQB1 alleles and absence of Asp 57 as susceptibility factors of IDDM in Finland. *Diabetes* 1991; **40**(12): 1640–1644.

Reynet C, Kahn CR. Rad: a member of the Ras family overexpressed in muscle of type II diabetic humans. *Science* 1993; **262**(5138): 1441–1444.

Riley WJ, MacLaren NK, Krischer J, Spillar RP, Silverstein JH, Schatz DA, Schwartz S, Malone J, Shah S, Vadheim C, et al. A prospective study of the development of diabetes in relatives of patients with insulin-dependent diabetes. *N Engl J Med* 1990; **323**: 1167–1172.

Rissanen J, Pihlajamaki J, Heikkinen S, Kekalainen P, Mykkanen L, Kuusisto J, Kolle A, Laakso M. New variants in the glycogen synthase gene (Gln71His, Met416Val) in patients with NIDDM from eastern Finland. *Diabetologia* 1997; **4011**: 1313–1319.

Samaras K, Campbell LV. The non-genetic determinants of central adiposity. *Int J Obes Relat Metab Disord* 1997; **21**(10): 839–845.

Schneider SH, Amorosa LF, Khachadurian AK, Ruderman NB. Studies on the mechanism of improved glucose control during regular exercise in type 2 (non-insulin-dependent) diabetes. *Diabetologia* 1984; **26**(5): 355–360.

Schoenle EJ, Molinari L, Bagot M, Semadeni S, Wiesendanger M. Epidemiology of IDDM in Switzerland. Increasing incidence rate and rural-urban differences in Swiss men born

1948–1972. *Diabetes Care* 1994; **17**(9): 955–960.

Scott FW, Mongeau R, Kardish M, Hatina G, Trick KD, Wojcinski Z. Diet can prevent diabetes in the BB rat. *Diabetes* 1985; **34**: 1059–1062.

Seidell JC, Han TS, Feskens EJ, Lean ME. Narrow hips and broad waist circumferences independently contribute to increased risk of non-insulin-dependent diabetes mellitus. *J Intern Med* 1997; **242**(5): 401–406.

Shimizu M, Kawazu S, Tomono S, Ohno T, Utsugi T, Kato N, Ishi C, Ito Y, Murata K. Age-related alteration of pancreatic beta-cell function. Increased proinsulin and proinsulin-to-insulin molar ratio in elderly, but not in obese, subjects without glucose intolerance. *Diabetes Care* 1996; **19**(1): 8–11.

Shimomura H, Sanke T, Ueda K, Hanabusa T, Sakagashira S, Nanjo K. A missense mutation of the muscle glycogen synthase gene (M416V) is associated with insulin resistance in the Japanese population. *Diabetologia* 1997; **40**(8): 947–952.

Siemiatycki J, Colle E, Campbell S, Dewar R, Aubert D, Belmonte MM. Incidence of IDDM in Montreal by ethnic group and by social class and comparisons with ethnic groups living elsewhere. *Diabetes* 1988; **37**: 1096–1102.

Skarfors ET, Selinus KI, Lithell HO. Risk factors for developing non-insulin dependent diabetes: a 10 year follow up of men in Uppsala. *BMJ* 1991; **303**(6805): 755–760.

Skolnick AA. First Type I diabetes prevention trials. *JAMA* 1997; **277**(14): 1101–1102.

Sonnenberg GE. The new classification and diagnostic criteria for diabetes mellitus: rationale and implications. *WMJ* 1998; **97**(3): 27–29.

Srikanta S, Ganda OP, Jackson RA, Gleason RE, Kaldany A, Garovoy MR, Milford EL, Carpenter CB, Soeldner JS, Eisenbarth GS. Type 1 diabetes mellitus in monozygotic twins: chronic progressive β-cell dysfunction. *Ann Int Med* 1983; **99**: 320–326.

Stoffers DA, Ferrer J, Clarke WL, Habener JF. Early-onset type-II diabetes mellitus (MODY4) linked to IPF1. *Nat Genet* 1997; **17**(2): 138–139.

Tarn AC, Thomas JM, Dean BM, Ingram D, Schwartz G, Bottazzo GF, Gale EA. Predicting insulin-dependent diabetes. *Lancet* 1988; **I**: 845–850.

Tattersal RB, Pyke DA. Diabetes in identical twins. *Lancet* 1972; **II**: 1120–1125.

Taylor R, Ram P, Zimmet P, Raper LR, Ringrose H. Physical activity and prevalence of diabetes in Melanesian and Indian men in Fiji. *Diabetologia* 1984; **27**(6): 578–582.

Thomson G, Robinson WP, Kuhner MK, Joe S, MacDonald MJ, Gottschall JL, Barbosa J, Rich SS, Bertrams J, Baur MP, et al. Genetic heterogeneity, modes of inheritance, and risk estimates for a joint study of Caucasians with insulin-dependent diabetes mellitus. *Am J Hum Genet* 1988; **43**(6): 799–816.

Todd JA. Genetics of type I diabetes. *Pathol Biol (Paris)* 1997; **45**(3): 219–227.

Todd JA, Bell JI, McDevitt HO. HLA-DQ beta gene contributes to susceptibility and resistance to insulin-dependent diabetes mellitus. *Nature* 1987; **329**(6140): 599–604.

Todd JA, Farrall M. Panning for gold: genome-wide scanning for linkage in type I diabetes. *Hum Mol Genet* 1996; **5**(Spec): 1443–1448.

Tonolo G, Melis MG, Ciccarese M, Secchi G, Atzeni MM, Li LS, Luthman H, Maioli M. Glucagon receptor Gly40Ser amino acid variant in Sardinian hypertensive non-insulin-dependent diabetic patients. Sardinian Diabetic Genetic Study Group (SDGSG). *Acta Diabetol* 1997; **34**(2): 75–76.

Undlien DE, Bennett ST, Todd JA, Akselsen HE, Ikaheimo I, Reijonen H, Knip M, Thorsby E, Ronningen KS. Insulin gene region-encoded susceptibility to IDDM maps upstream of the insulin gene. *Diabetes* 1995; **44**(6): 620–625.

Ura S, Araki E, Kishikawa H, Shirotani T, Todaka M, Isami S, Shimoda S, Yoshimura R, Matsuda K, Motoyoshi S, et al. Molecular scanning of the insulin receptor substrate-1 (IRS-1) gene in Japanese patients with NIDDM: identification of five novel polymorphisms. *Diabetologia* 1996; **39**(5): 600–608.

Valdez R, Athens MA, Thompson GH, Bradshaw BS, Stern MP. Birthweight and adult healthy outcomes in a biethnic populations in the USA. *Diabetologia* 1994; **37**(6): 624–631.

van den Ouwenland JMW, Lemkes HHPJ, Ruitenbeek W, Sandkujl L, deVijlder M, Struyvenberg PA, van de Kamp JJ, Maassen JA. Mutation in mitochondrial tRNALeu(UUR) gene in a large pedigree with maternally transmitted type II diabetes mellitus and deafness. *Nature Genet* 1992; **1**: 368–371.

Vela M, Adorno D, Longo A, Papola F, Maccarone D, Centis D, Raponi MP, Candela A, Campea L, Orsini M, et al. HLA typing data on 100 type I (insulin-dependent) diabetic patients from central Italy show a negative association with DR5 rather than with DR2. *Clin Immunol Immunopathol* 1987; **45**(1): 143–146.

Velho G, Froguel PH. Genetic determinants of non-insulin-dependent diabetes mellitus: strategies and recent results. *Diabete Metab* 1997; **23**(1): 7–17.

Vionnet N, Stoffel M, Takeda J, Yasuda K, Bell G, Zouali M, Lesage S, Velho G, Iris F, Passa P, et al. Nonsense mutation in the glucokinase gene causes early-onset non-insulin-dependent diabetes mellitus. *Nature* 1992; **356**: 721–722.

Virtanen SM, Jaakkola L, Rasanen L, Ylonen K, Aro A, Lounamaa R, Akerblom HK, Tuomilehto J. Nitrate and nitrite intake and the risk for type 1 diabetes in Finnish children. Childhood Diabetes in Finland Study Group. *Diabet Med* 1994a; **11**(7): 656–662.

Virtanen SM, Saukkonen T, Savilahti E, Ylonen K, Rasanen L, Aro A, Knip M, Tuomilehto J, Akerblom HK. Diet, cow's milk protein antibodies, and the risk of IDDM in Finnish children. Childhood Diabetes in Finland Study Group. *Diabetologia* 1994b; **37**(4): 381–387.

Vreugdenhil GR, Gelluk A, Ottenhoff TH, Melchers WJ, Roep BO, Galama JM. Molecular mimicry in diabetes mellitus: the homologous domain in coxsackie B virus protein 2C and islet autoantigen GAD65 is highly conserved in the coxsackie B-like enteroviruses and binds to the diabetes associated with HLA-DR3 molecule. *Diabetologia* 1998; **41**(1): 40–46.

Wilson PW, Anderson KM, Kannel WB. Epidemiology of diabetes mellitus in the elderly. The Framingham Study. *Am J Med* 1986; **80**(5A): 3–9.

Yamagata K, Furata H, Oda N, Kaisaki PJ, Menzel S, Cox NJ, Fajans SS, Signorini S, Stoffel M, Bell GI. Mutations in the hepatocyte nuclear factor-4α gene in maturity-onset diabetes of the young (MODY1). *Nature* 1996a; **384**: 458–460.

Yamagata K, Oda N, Kaisaki PJ, Menzel S, Furuta H, Vaxillaire M, Southam L, Cox RD, Lathrop GM, Boriraj VV. Mutations in the hepatocyte nuclear factor-1α gene in maturity-onset diabetes of the young (MODY3). *Nature* 1996b; **384**: 455–458.

Yki-Jarvinen H. Evidence for a primary role of insulin resistance in the pathogenesis of type 2 diabetes. *Ann Med* 1990; **22**(3): 197–200.

Yoon JW, Onodera T, Notkins AL. Virus-induced diabetes mellitus. XV. Beta cell damage and insulin-dependent hyperglycemia in mice infected with coxsackie virus B4. *J Exp Med* 1978; **148**(4): 1068–1080.

2

COMPLICATIONS OF
DIABETES

Both type 1 and type 2 diabetes are accompanied by long-term microvascular or macrovascular complications that can result in serious morbidity and premature mortality. It is the complications of diabetes that contribute to the enormous costs, both economic and personal, that are associated with this disease. In general, symptoms of these complications develop years after the emergence of overt hyperglycemia (Foster, 1991), suggesting a window for therapeutic prevention strategies.

MICROVASCULAR COMPLICATIONS

Diabetic microangiopathy is characterized by an uneven thickening of the interior walls of small arterioles, leading to disruption of local circulation in the kidney, retina, and peripheral and autonomic nerves (McMillan, 1997). Consequently, microangiopathy is manifested clinically by the development of retinopathy and nephropathy, and is also believed to contribute to neuropathy in diabetic patients. Although the mechanisms underlying the development of microangiopathy have not been definitively defined, these vascular changes appear to be preceded by an increase in capillary pressure and capillary permeability to albumin, presumably due to hyperglycemia-induced metabolic disturbances (Valensi et al., 1998; Jaap et al., 1996; Jaap et al., 1993; Sandeman et al., 1992). Metabolic disturbances implicated in this process include the increased glycation of proteins, increased flux through the polyol pathway via aldose reductase, and the generation of oxidative stress (Cameron & Cotter, 1997). Glucose-induced activation of protein kinase C (PKC) has also been implicated in increased vascular permeability, cell proliferation, and resulting abnormal retinal and renal hemodynamics. Injury resulting from the increase in microvascular pressure may then contribute to abnormalities in vasodilation and autoregulatory capacity, and eventually damage to peripheral tissues (Tooke, 1995).

Recently, data from the Diabetes Control and Complications Trial (DCCT) provided the first evidence that genetic factors may also play a role in the development of nephropathy and the severity of retinopathy in patients with type 1 diabetes (DCCT Research Group, 1997). The UKPDS also found that genetic factors may contribute to the progression of nephropathy in patients with type 2 diabetes (Dudley et al., 1995). Further research in this area will be necessary to determine the contribution of genetics to these microvascular complications.

Retinopathy

Diabetic retinopathy is the leading cause of vision loss among working-age individuals in developed countries (Skolnick, 1997). Previous studies have reported that approximately 19% of patients with type 1 diabetes and 24% of patients with type 2 diabetes develop retinopathy three to four years after disease onset (Klein et al., 1984a, 1984b). As the frequency of retinopathy increases with diabetes duration, it has been estimated that nearly all individuals with type 1 diabetes, and 60% of individuals with type 2 diabetes, develop this complication after 20 years. In general, however, retinopathy tends to occur early in the disease process and is often the first microvascular complication to become evident, as its effects can be directly observed with opthalmoscopic examination.

In its initial stages, retinopathy is characterized by increased capillary permeability, capillary closures, microaneurysms, and small retinal hemorrhages. The development of soft exudates (infarcts of the retinal nerve) and hard exudates (retinal lipid deposits) may also occur. Collectively, these lesions are often referred to as "simple" (or "background") lesions. Retinopathy may then progress to the appearance of "proliferative" lesions, which include the development of new blood vessels, scarring, vitreal hemorrhaging, and retinal detachment. Due to evidence that hyperglycemia is strongly associated with the development of retinopathy, it has been suggested that metabolic disturbances may result in functional changes in retinal blood vessels and the eventual appearance of lesions and angiogenesis (Klein & Klein, 1997). However, the mechanism underlying these changes is unclear.

Table 2.1 - Early Treatment Diabetic Retinopathy Study Classification System: examples of graded characteristics.

Characteristics Graded in Multiple Photographic Fields	Characteristics Graded only in Field 1 (Optic Disk)
• Microaneurysms • Hemorrhages and/or microaneurysms • Drusen • Hard exudates • Soft exudates • Intraretinal microvascular abnormalities • Venous abnormalities • Arteriolar abnormalities • Arteriovenous nicking • New vessels on the retinal surface • Dilated tips of new vessels • Fibrous proliferations • Plane of proliferation • Preretinal hemorrhage • Vitreous hemorrhage • Retinal elevation • Scars of prior photocoagulation	• New vessels • Dilated tips of new vessels • Fibrous proliferations • Plane of proliferation • Papillary swelling **Characteristics Graded only in Field 2 (Macula)** • Hard exudate rings • Posterior vitreous detachment • Retinal thickening • Size of thickened area • Maximum thickness of thickened area • Cystoid spaces • Clinically significant macular edema

The severity of diabetic retinopathy can be assessed using the Early Treatment Diabetic Retinopathy Study (ETDRS) grading system, which is a extended version of the Modified Airlie House classification (Early Treatment Diabetic Retinopathy Study Research Group, 1991a). With this system, seven-field stereoscopic fundus photographs of the eyes are analyzed for characteristic abnormalities, which are graded separately on a numerical scale. These abnormalities can be graded either in multiple photographic fields or in single fields on the optic disc or macula (Table 2.1). A single severity level can then be calculated from the individual scores (Early Treatment Diabetic Retinopathy Study Research Group, 1991b). An alternative measure to assess the severity of retinopathy is fluorescein fundus angiography, which provides a detailed examination of the retinal capillary bed (Early Treatment Diabetic Retinopathy Study Research Group, 1991c). Finally, functional abnormalities may be evaluated with tests of visual acuity, color vision, perimetry, and contrast sensitivity.

The development and progression of retinopathy are associated with increased levels of advanced glycation end products (AGEs), which are thought to mediate damage to blood vessels in the retina as well as other organs in diabetes (Ruggiero-Lopez et al., 1997; Beisswenger et al., 1995). In addition, vascular endothelial growth factor (VEGF) is consistently elevated in the retinas of patients with diabetes, and appears to contribute to both increased capillary permeability and retinal angiogenesis (Lu et al., 1998). AGEs have been shown to induce the expression of VEGF in diabetic retinas (Hirata et al., 1997; Murata et al., 1997), suggesting a potential mechanism for their role in the progression of retinopathy. AGEs may also contribute to the generation of oxidative stress and DNA damage (Wautier et al., 1994). Activity of aldose reductase, the rate-limiting enzyme in the polyol pathway converting glucose to sorbitol, has also been correlated with the degree of diabetic retinopathy (Nishimura et al., 1997). It has been suggested that the accumulation of metabolites from this pathway (sorbitol and fructose) may enhance AGE production and the exacerbation of vascular damage in peripheral tissues (Tomlinson et al., 1992; Brownlee, 1992).

Based on what has been learned about factors contributing to the pathogenesis of retinopathy, several strategies to prevent or slow its progression have been proposed. Intensive insulin treatment achieving a mean reduction in glycated hemoglobin (HbA_{1c}) of approximately 1.7% has been shown to reduce the adjusted mean risk of retinopathy by 76% and to slow its progression by 54% in patients with type 1 diabetes, as compared to conventional therapy (DCCT Research Group, 1993). The development of retinopathy was also reduced in patients with type 2 diabetes receiving intensive insulin therapy (Ohkubo et al., 1995). Most recently, the United Kingdom Prospective Diabetes Study (UKPDS) demonstrated a reduced relative risk for the progression of retinopathy in type 2 diabetic patients receiving intensive therapy in comparison to conventional treatment (UKPDS Group, 1998). However, the level of metabolic control achieved in the DCCT may not be easily achieved in clinical practice (Klein et al., 1996).

Other approaches aimed at reducing the development of retinopathy include angiotensin-converting enzyme inhibition (e.g., captopril), inhibition of AGE formation (e.g., aminoguanidine), inhibition of action at the AGE receptor binding site (RAGE), and inhibition of VEGF-activated protein kinase C (Skolnick, 1997). Several aldose reductase inhibitors have also been examined as therapies for retinopathy, although they have not yet demonstrated the ability to prevent or reduce the progression of retinopathy in clinical trials.

Surgical interventions for diabetic retinopathy include photocoagulation and vitrectomy. Panretinal photocoagulation involves the delivery of 1500 to 2000 laser burns around the central retina, in order to reduce the abnormal growth of new blood vessels. This technique has been shown to reduce severe visual loss in patients with proliferative retinopathy; however, it also carries the risk of moderate losses in visual field and visual acuity (Diabetic Retinopathy Study Group, 1981; Early Treatment Diabetic Retinopathy Research Study Group, 1985). Vitrectomy entails the removal of vitreous hemorrhages or the transection of fibers that cause retinal detachment. A follow-up study of this procedure in patients with severe diabetic vitreous hemorrhage demonstrated significantly better recovery of visual acuity with early vitrectomy (in comparison to a deferral of one year) for patients with type 1, but not type 2, diabetes (Diabetic Retinopathy Vitrectomy Study Research Group, 1985). The major adverse effects associated with this procedure are iatrogenic retinal detachments and neovascular glaucoma, which could result in total visual loss (Klein and Klein, 1997). Thus, fully safe and effective surgical options are not currently available, and the ultimate goal of therapy for diabetic retinopathy is the inhibition of its development, and the avoidance of lesions requiring surgical intervention.

Nephropathy

Nephropathy accounts for approximately one third of all cases of end-stage renal disease in the U.S., and is a major cause of morbidity and mortality in patients with diabetes (Kobrin, 1998). The syndrome is characterized by a variety of glomerular lesions and other structural abnormalities, as well as functional changes in the kidney. Increased plasma flow and capillary pressure have been noted as early events in the development of nephropathy. These altered circulatory conditions probably result in part from impaired vasculature autoregulation, which is secondary to the metabolic disorder. Nephropathy results from increased glomerular filtration, resulting cell damage, and thickening of the basement membrane. Evidence for this pathway has been documented in studies showing that glomerular hyperfiltration develops soon after the onset of diabetes, and remains elevated until overt nephropathy appears (Nelson et al., 1997). Following this stage, in which glomerular hyperfiltration is the only obvious functional change, is a progression to microproteinuria (microalbuminuria) in about 20–45% of patients (Mogensen et al., 1992; Niazy et al., 1987; Andersen et al., 1983). Macroproteinuria (albuminuria) then develops among these patients at a rate of 11% per year (DCCT Research Group, 1995). Macroproteinuria precedes a steady decline in glomerular filtration and renal function (Nelson et al., 1996; Deckert et al., 1991). Once established, nephropathy progresses to end-stage renal failure over a period averaging about seven years, although the individual course can vary substantially (Grenfell and Watkins, 1986). At this stage, treatment options include dialysis or kidney transplantation. Factors associated with the progression of nephropathy include high levels of AGEs, hypertension, hyperglycemia, and high cholesterol (Ravid et al., 1998; Mehler et al., 1997; Beisswenger et al., 1995).

The progression of diabetic nephropathy can be monitored with the evaluation of urine albumin values and the rate of glomerular filtration. Microproteinuria is defined as an albumin excretion rate of 30–300 mg/day (Mogensen et al., 1995), and marks the onset of "incipient nephropathy." Progression to "clinical diabetic nephropathy" is characterized by the development of macroproteinuria, or an albumin excretion rate of greater than 300 mg/day. Macroproteinuria can also be assessed with dipstick measurements. Glomerular filtration rate is a standard measure of renal function, and can be assessed via the clearance of various markers which are filtered by the kidney (Gaspari et al., 1997). Once nephropathy is established, the rate of glomerular filtration generally declines at a rate of 10 ml/min per year (Selby et al., 1990).

Although no direct anti-nephropathic therapies are currently available, substantial evidence has accumulated that some antihypertensive compounds can slow, or even prevent, the progression of nephropathy (Crepaldi et al., 1998; Ahmad et al., 1997; Sawicki, 1997; Ravid et al., 1996; Microalbuminuria Captopril Study Group, 1996). In particular, certain angiotensin-converting enzyme inhibitors (ACE inhibitors) and calcium channel blockers have demonstrated nephroprotective properties beyond their blood pressure-lowering effects. It has been suggested that in addition to reducing pressure on the glomerular arterioles, these compounds may work directly on renal cells to reduce basement membrane alterations (Goldfarb and Henrich, 1998; Parving et al., 1996). Intensive anti-hyperglycemic therapy has also been shown to markedly reduce the risk of nephropathy in type 1 and type 2 diabetic patients (UKPDS Group, 1998; Bojestig et al., 1996; Ohkubo et al., 1995; DCCT Research Group, 1993).

Neuropathy

Neuropathy is responsible for substantial morbidity in the diabetic population, and can result in life-threatening complications. There are several distinct manifestations of neuropathy, including peripheral polyneuropathy, autonomic neuropathy, and mononeuropathy. Peripheral polyneuropathy is the most common form, and is associated with numbness, paresthesia, and pain in the periphery. The secondary development of ulcers and gangrene in the lower extremities is all too common in patients afflicted with this complication. The symptoms of peripheral polyneuropathy are progressive, and their severity correlates with the degree of impaired glycemic control (Partanen et al., 1995). Autonomic neuropathy is predominantly characterized by gastrointestinal symptoms, including gastroparesis, nocturnal diarrhea, and constipation. Orthostatic hypotension and frank syncope may also occur. Mononeuropathy (or focal neuropathy) tends to affect single nerves, most commonly the third, sixth, or seventh cranial nerves, and primarily appears to be a vascular effect on large nerve fiber bundles (Thomas, 1997). Unlike the other neuropathies, mononeuropathic symptoms often reverse spontaneously.

Although its pathogenesis is not clearly understood, the development and severity of diabetic neuropathy is strongly associated with microangiopathy, particularly the thickening of basement membranes and endothelial hyperplasia (Malik, 1997). The involvement of reduced nerve blood flow in the development of neuropathy is supported by evidence that vasodilator treatment prevents or reverses defects in nerve conduction velocity *in vivo* (reviewed in Cameron & Cotter, 1997). Like other microvascular complications, the severity of neuropathy is proportional to the level of hyperglycemia (Allen et al., 1997). Metabolic disturbances associated with hyperglycemia, such as increased aldose reductase activity, the formation of AGEs, or both, have also been associated with deleterious effects on nerve conduction velocity in animal models.

There are several methods to evaluate the progression of diabetic neuropathy, including vibratory, thermal, or monofilament testing for the assessment of large-fiber symmetric polyneuropathy, and cardiovascular reflex testing (heart rate variability or Valsalva maneuver) for the assessment of autonomic neuropathy (Hirsch, 1996). More invasive methods include the evaluation of nerve conduction velocity or sural nerve biopsy (Thomas, 1997).

The established strategy for the prevention of diabetic neuropathy is to strive to achieve near normal ("tight") glycemic control. The DCCT showed that the occurrence of overt neuropathy was reduced by 60% in type 1 patients receiving intensive insulin treatment (DCCT Research Group, 1993). Meticulous glycemic control was also associated with improved nerve conduction velocity and vibration perception thresholds in patients with type 2 diabetes (UKPDS Group, 1998; Ohkubo et al., 1995). In addition, aldose reductase inhibitors have demonstrated a positive impact on nerve conduction velocity and axonal regeneration in clinical trials, although effects were modest (Macleod et al., 1992; van Gerven et al., 1992; Sima et al., 1988). Treatments for symptoms of peripheral neuropathy include analgesics and tricyclic antidepressants for pain. Erythromycin and metoclopramide are used for symptomatic gastroparesis (Clark & Lee, 1995).

MACROVASCULAR COMPLICATIONS

Diabetic macroangiopathy is characterized by atherosclerosis in coronary, peripheral, and cerebral arteries, clinically manifested by ischemic heart disease, peripheral vascular disease, and stroke. It is a leading cause of mortality in the diabetic population; recent estimates indicate that coronary artery disease and stroke account for 50% and 15% of deaths in type 2 patients, respectively (Nathan et al., 1997). It is well established that patients with diabetes develop atherosclerosis earlier and at a more rapid rate than non-diabetic individuals. Moreover, the risk of cardiovascular disease in diabetic patients is two to five times greater than in individuals without diabetes (Meigs et al., 1997; World Health Organization, 1994; Panzram, 1987). To a certain extent, differences in prevalence may be due to the association of diabetes with known risk factors for atherosclerosis, including hypertension, lipid abnormalities, and obesity (i.e., Syndrome X). However, these factors cannot entirely account for the accelerated vascular disease observed in this population.

Although the precise mechanism is not established, it is clear that AGEs play a role in the pathogenesis of macroangiopathy. An association between diabetes and increased levels of glycated low density lipoproteins (LDLs) has consistently been reported (Sobenin et al., 1996; Yegin et al., 1995; Cohen et al., 1993). Glycated LDL is rapidly internalized by macrophages (Lopes-Virella et al., 1988), resulting in the formation of foam cells, an early characteristic of atherosclerosis (Brown & Goldstein, 1983). Moreover, glycated LDL is more susceptible to oxidative modification (Yegin et al., 1995; Bellomo et al., 1995); oxidation of LDL may contribute to macroangiopathy since oxidized forms of LDL are more atherogenic than parent LDL (Bellomo et al., 1995). Glycated LDL also increases platelet aggregation, which may accelerate the development of atherosclerotic fibrous plaques (Takeda et al., 1992).

Preventive strategies for macroangiopathy include those used to reduce the risk of atherosclerosis in non-diabetic patients, such as diet, exercise, lipid-lowering compounds, anti-platelet agents, and antihypertensive medications. In addition, therapy to achieve meticulous glycemic control has been recommended (Colwell, 1997). In contrast to the clear benefits observed for microangiopathy, however, the role of glycemic control in the prevention of macroangiopathy is unclear. An 8-year study conducted by the University Group Diabetes Program (UGDP) reported that intensive insulin therapy did not slow the rate of progression to major cardiovascular endpoints in patients with type 2 diabetes (University Group Diabetes Program, 1970). Moreover, the use of agents to enhance metabolic control (the sulfonylurea tolbutamide and the biguanide phenformin) was associated with an increase in the incidence of major cardiovascular events compared to diet-only-treated patients in this study. A more recent study suggested that intensive blood glucose control may slow the development of atherosclerosis in patients with type 1 diabetes, on the basis of improved arterial wall stiffness and thickness associated with improved glycemic control (Jensen-Urstad et al., 1996). The DCCT failed to show a relationship between improved glycemic control and macrovascular-related outcomes in type 1 patients. Likewise, the 11-year results of the UKPDS did not support a beneficial effect of strict glycemic control on the development of macrovascular disease in type 2 patients. The UKPDS did not however, report an excess of cardiovascular events associated with biguanide therapy (metformin in this study), as was the case for biguanide therapy in the UGDP study. A somewhat higher event rate relative to the diet-only-treated group was seen for the sulfonylurea-treated patients (UKPDS Group, 1998).

DYSLIPIDEMIA

As noted previously, dyslipidemia contributes to the high risk of atherosclerosis and heart disease in diabetic patients. The profile of dyslipidemia in patients with both type 1 and type 2 diabetes is characterized by increased levels of triglycerides, smaller (i.e., more atherogenic) LDL particle size, and decreased levels of high-density lipoprotein (HDL; Laakso et al., 1997; Hirano et al., 1996). This profile has also been observed in non-diabetic patients with insulin resistance, suggesting that insulin resistance is responsible for this dyslipidemic pattern (Salonen et al., 1998). Worsening glycemic control itself results in an exacerbation of dyslipidemia in diabetic patients (Laakso, 1997). In addition, reduced receptor-mediated clearance of LDL has been linked to the formation of AGEs *in vivo*, providing a potential connection between metabolic disturbances and lipid abnormalities.

Hypertriglyceridemia is a strong, independent predictor of coronary heart disease, and small LDL particles have demonstrated an association with the development of nephropathy (Hirano et al., 1996; Assmann et al., 1996). Thus, improved control of dyslipidemia could potentially reduce both microvascular and macrovascular complications. As a means of achieving better control of the dyslipidemia, exercise and a low-cholesterol diet are recommended, followed by therapy to achieve good glycemic control. Previous studies have demonstrated reductions in triglycerides and hyperinsulinemia in diabetic patients following diet and exercise interventions (Barnard et al., 1994; Barnard et al., 1992). In addition, improved glycemic control was associated with improvements in dyslipidemia in patients with both type 1 and type 2 diabetes (Perez et al., 1997; Romano et al., 1997). In those patients with dyslipidemia who do not respond to diet and exercise, lipid-lowering drugs may be indicated. The statins, or 3-hydroxy-3-methylglutaryl coenzyme A reductase inhibitors, have become the treatment of choice in first-line drug therapy for diabetic dyslipidemia (Garg, 1998). A recent overview reported that statin therapy significantly reduces total and LDL cholesterol, as well as the risk of stroke and mortality due to cardiovascular disease, in the general population of hyperlipidemic patients (Herbert et al., 1997). However, large, well-controlled trials of lipid-lowering therapy in diabetic patients are necessary to establish similar benefits of these therapies for the diabetic population.

CONCLUSIONS

The microvascular and macrovascular complications of diabetes are responsible for substantial morbidity and mortality in this patient population. However, an increased understanding of the pathogenesis of these complications has established the foundation for more effective treatment approaches. The landmark results of the DCCT and UKPDS provided the first breakthrough, demonstrating the long-suspected relationship between glycemic control and the reduction of microvascular complications. Increasing evidence implicating AGEs and the aldose reductase pathway in the development of complications has provided additional therapeutic targets. The development of more direct treatment strategies for diabetic complications represents a fundamental change in the therapeutic approach to diabetes, and has the potential to expand options to include the prevention or reduction of the devastating consequences of this disease.

References

Ahmad J, Siddiqui MA, Ahmad H. Effective postponement of diabetic nephropathy with enalapril in normotensive type 2 diabetic patients with microalbuminuria. *Diabetes Care* 1997; **20**(10): 1576–1581.

Allen C, Shen G, Palta M, Lotz B, Jacobson R, D'Alessio D. Long-term hyperglycemia is related to peripheral nerve changes at a diabetes duration of 4 years. The Wisconsin Diabetes Registry. *Diabetes Care* 1997; **20**(7): 1154–1158.

Andersen AR, Christiansen JS, Andersen JK, Kreiner S, Deckert T. Diabetic nephropathy in type 1 (insulin-dependent) diabetes: an epidemiological study. *Diabetologia* 1983; **25**(6): 496–501.

Assmann G, Schulte H, von Eckardstein A. Hypertriglyceridemia and elevated lipoprotein(a) are risk factors for major coronary events in middle-aged men. *Am J Cardiol* 1996; **77**(14): 1179–1184.

Barnard RJ, Jung T, Inkeles SB. Diet and exercise in the treatment of NIDDM. The need for early emphasis. *Diabetes Care* 1994; **17**(12): 1469–1472.

Barnard RJ, Ugianskis EJ, Martin DA, Inkeles SB. Role of diet and exercise in the management of hyperinsulinemia and associated atherosclerotic risk factors. *Am J Cardiol* 1992; **69**(5): 440–444.

Beisswenger PJ, Makita Z, Curphey TJ, Moore LL, Jean S, Brinck-Johnsen T, Bucala R, Vlassara H. Formation of immunochemical advanced glycosylation end products precedes and correlates with early manifestations of renal and retinal disease in diabetes. *Diabetes* 1995; **44**(7): 824–829.

Bellomo G, Maggi E, Poli M, Agosta FG, Bollati P, Finardi G. Autoantibodies against oxidatively modified low-density lipoproteins in NIDDM. *Diabetes* 1995; **44**(1): 60–66.

Bojestig M, Arnqvist HJ, Karlberg BE, Ludvigsson J. Glycemic control and prognosis in type 1 diabetic patients with microalbuminuria. *Diabetes Care* 1996; **19**(4): 313–317.

Brown MS, Goldstein JL. Lipoprotein metabolism in the macrophage: implications for cholesterol deposition in atherosclerosis. *Annu Rev Biochem* 1983; **52**: 223–261.

Brownlee M. Glycation products and the pathogenesis of diabetic complications. *Diabetes Care* 1992; **15**: 1835–1843.

Cameron NE, Cotter MA. Metabolic and vascular factors in the pathogenesis of diabetic neuropathy. *Diabetes* 1997; **46**(Suppl 2): S31–S37.

Clark CM, Lee DA. Prevention and treatment of the complications of diabetes mellitus. *N Engl J Med* 1995; **332**(18): 1210–1217.

Cohen MP, Lautenslager G, Shea E. Glycated LDL concentrations in non-diabetic and diabetic subjects measured with monoclonal antibodies reactive with glycated apolipoprotein B epitopes. *Eur J Clin Chem Clin Biochem* 1993; **31**(11): 707–713.

Colwell JA. Pharmacological strategies to prevent macrovascular disease in NIDDM. *Diabetes* 1997; **46**(Suppl 2): 131–134.

Crepaldi G, Carta Q, Deferrari G, Mangili R, Navalesi R, Santeusanio F, Spalluto A, Vanasia A, Villa GM, Nosadini R. Effects of lisinopril and nifedipine on the progression to overt albuminuria in IDDM patients with incipient nephropathy and normal blood pressure. The Italian Microalbuminuria Study Group in IDDM. *Diabetes Care* 1998; **21**(1): 104–110.

DCCT Research Group. The effect of intensive treatment of diabetes on the development and progression of long-term complications in insulin-dependent diabetes mellitus. *N Engl J Med* 1993; **329**(14): 977–986.

DCCT Research Group. Effect of intensive therapy on the development and progression of diabetic nephropathy in the Diabetes Control and Complications Trial. *Kidney Int* 1995; **47**(6): 1703–1720.

DCCT Research Group. Clustering of long-term complications in families with diabetes in the Diabetes Control and Complications Trial. *Diabetes* 1997; **46**(11): 1829–1839.

Deckert T, Feldt-Rasmussen B, Borch-Johnsen K, Jensen T, Kofoed-Enevoldsen A, Mathiesen ER. Natural history of diabetic complications: early detection and progression. *Diabet Med* 1991; **8**(Spec No): 33–37.

Diabetic Retinopathy Study Group. Photocoagulation treatment of proliferative diabetic retinopathy: clinical application of Diabetic Retinopathy Study (DRS) findings. DRS Report No. 8. *Opthalmology* 1981; **88**: 583–600.

Diabetic Retinopathy Vitrectomy Study Research Group. Early vitrectomy for severe vitreous hemorrhage in diabetic retinopathy: two-year results of a randomized trial. DRVS Report No. 2. *Arch Opthalmol* 1985; **92**: 492–502.

Dudley CR, Keavney B, Stratton IM, Turner RC, Ratcliffe PJ. UK Prospective Diabetes Study XV: relationship of renin-angiotensin system gene polymorphisms with microalbuminuria in NIDDM. *Kidney Int* 1995; **48**(6): 1907–1911.

Early Treatment Diabetic Retinopathy Study Research Group. Photocoagulation for diabetic macular edema. *Arch Opthalmol* 1985; **103**: 1796–1806.

Early Treatment Diabetic Retinopathy Study Research Group. Grading diabetic retinopathy from stereoscopic color fundus photographs–an extension of the modified Airlie House Classification. ETDRS Report No. 10. *Ophthalmology* 1991a; **98**(Suppl 5): 786–806.

Early Treatment Diabetic Retinopathy Study Research Group. Fundus photographic risk factors for progression of diabetic retinopathy. ETDRS Report No. 12. *Opthalmology* 1991b; **98**(Suppl 5): 823–833.

Early Treatment Diabetic Retinopathy Study Research Group. Classification of diabetic retinopathy from fluorescein angiograms. ETDRS Report No. 11. *Opthalmology* 1991c; **98**(Suppl 5): 807–822.

Foster DW. Diabetes mellitus. In Wilson JD, Braunwald E, Isselbacher KJ, Petersdorf RG, Martin JB, Fauci AS, Root RK (eds) *Harrison's Principles of Internal Medicine, 12th edition.* New York: McGraw-Hill, 1991, pp. 1739–1758.

Garg A. Treatment of diabetic dyslipidemia. *Am J Cardiol* 1998; **81**(4A): 47–51.

Gaspari F, Perico N, Remuzzi G. Measurement of glomerular filtration rate. *Kidney Int Suppl* 1997; **63**: S151–S154.

Goldfarb S, Henrich WL. Update in nephrology. *Ann Intern Med* 1998; **128**(1): 49–55.

Grenfell A, Watkins PJ. Clinical diabetic nephropathy: natural history and complications. *Clin Endocrinol Metab* 1986; **15**(4): 783–805.

Herbert PR, Gaziano JM, Chan KS, Hennekens CH. Cholesterol lowering with statin drugs, risk of stroke, and total mortality. An overview of randomized trials. *JAMA* 1997; **278**(4): 313–321.

Hirano T, Naito H, Kurokawa M, Ebara T, Nagano S, Adachi M, Yoshino G. High prevalence of small LDL particles in non-insulin-dependent diabetic patients with nephropathy. *Atherosclerosis* 1996; **123**(1–2): 57–72.

Hirata C, Nakano K, Nakamura N, Kitagawa Y, Shigeta H, Hasegawa G, Ogata M, Ikeda T, Sawa H, Nakamura K, et al. Advanced glycation end products induce expression of vascular endothelial growth factor by retinal Muller cells. *Biochem Biophys Res Commun* 1997; **236**(3): 712–715.

Hirsch IB. Surveillance for complications of diabetes: don't wait for symptoms before intervening. *Postgrad Med* 1996; **99**(3): 147–155.

Jaap AJ, Shore AC, Gartside IB, Gample J, Tooke JE. Increased microvascular fluid permeability in young type 1 (insulin-dependent) diabetic patients. *Diabetologia* 1993; **36**(7): 648–652.

Jaap AJ, Shore AC, Tooke JE. Differences in microvascular fluid permeability between long-duration type 1 (insulin-dependent) diabetic patients with and without significant microangiopathy. *Clin Sci (Colch)* 1996; **90**(2): 113–117.

Jensen-Urstad KJ, Reichard PG, Rosfors JS, Lindblad LE, Jensen-Urstad MT. Early atherosclerosis is retarded by improved long-term blood glucose control in patients with IDDM. *Diabetes* 1996; **45**(9): 1253–1258.

Klein R, Klein BEK. Diabetic eye disease. *Lancet* 1997; **350**: 197–204.

Klein R, Klein BEK, Moss SE, Cruickshanks KJ. The medical management of hyperglycemia over a 10-year period in people with diabetes. *Diabetes Care* 1996; **19**: 744–750.

Klein R, Klein BEK, Moss SE, Davis MD, DeMets DL. The Wisconsin Epidemiologic Study of Diabetic Retinopathy, II: prevalence and risk of diabetic retinopathy when age at diagnosis is less than 30 years. *Arch Opthalmol* 1984a; **102**: 520–526.

Klein R, Klein BEK, Moss SE, Davis MD, DeMets DL. The Wisconsin Epidemiologic Study of Diabetic Retinopathy, III: prevalence and risk of diabetic retinopathy when age at diagnosis is 30 or more years. *Arch Opthalmol* 1984b; **102**: 527–532.

Kobrin SM. Diabetic nephropathy. *Dis Mon* 1998; **44**(5): 214–234.

Laakso M. Dyslipidemia, morbidity, and mortality in non-insulin-dependent diabetes mellitus. Lipoproteins and coronary heart disease in non-insulin-dependent diabetes mellitus. *J Diabetes Complications* 1997; **11**(2): 137–141.

Lopes-Virella MF, Klein RI, Lyons TJ, Stevenson HC, Wiztum JL. Glycosylation of LDL enhances cholesterol ester synthesis in human monocyte-derived macrophages. *Diabetes* 1988; **37**: 550–557.

Lu M, Kuroki M, Amano S, Tolentino M, Keough K, Kim I, Bucala R, Adamis AP. Advanced glycation end products increase retinal vascular endothelial growth factor expression. *J Clin Invest* 1998; **101**(6): 1219–1224.

Macleod AF, Boulton AJ, Owens DR, Van Rooy P, van Gerven JM, Macrury S, Scarpello JH, Segers O, Heoller SR, Van Der Veen EA. A multicenter trial of the aldose-reductase inhibitor tolrestat, in patients with symptomatic diabetic peripheral neuropathy. North European Tolrestat Study Group. *Diabete Metab* 1992; **18**(1): 14–20.

Malik RA. The pathology of human diabetic neuropathy. *Diabetes* 1997; **46**(Suppl 2): 50–53.

McMillan DE. Development of vascular complications in diabetes. *Vasc Med* 1997; **2**(2): 132–142.

Mehler PS, Jeffers BW, Estacio R, Schrier RW. Associations of hypertension and complications in non-insulin-dependent diabetes mellitus. *Am J Hypertens* 1997; **10**(2): 152–161.

Meigs JB, Singer DE, Sullivan LM, Dukes KA, D'Agostino RB, Nathan DM, Wagner EH, Kaplan SH, Greenfield S. Metabolic control and prevalent cardiovascular disease in non-insulin-dependent diabetes mellitus (NIDDM): the NIDDM Patients Outcome Research Team. *Am J Med* 1997; **102**(1): 38–47.

Microalbuminuria Captopril Study Group. Captopril reduces the risk of nephropathy in IDDM patients with microalbuminuria. *Diabetologia* 1996; **39**(5): 587–593.

Mogensen CE, Damsgaard EM, Froland A, Nielsen S, de Fine Oliverius N, Schmitz A. Microalbuminuria in non-insulin-dependent diabetes. *Clin Nephrol* 1992; **38**(Suppl 1): S28–S39.

Mogensen CE, Vestbo E, Poulsen PL, Christiansen C, Damsgaard EM, Eiskjaer H, Froland A, Hansen KW, Nielsen S, Pedersen MM. Microalbuminuria and potential confounders. A review and some observations on variability of urinary albumin excretion. *Diabetes Care* 1995; **18**(4): 572–581.

Murata T, Nagai R, Ishibashi T, Inomuta H, Ikeda K, Horiuchi S. The relationship between accumulation of advanced glycation end products and expression of vascular endothelial growth factor in human diabetic retinas. *Diabetologia* 1997; **40**(7): 764–769.

Nathan DM, Meigs J, Singer DE. The epidemiology of cardiovascular disease in type 2 diabetes mellitus: how sweet it is... or is it? *Lancet* 1997; **350**(Suppl 1): 4–9.

Nelson RG, Bennett PH, Beck GJ, Tan M, Knowler WC, Mitch WE, Hirschman GH, Myers BD. Development and progression of renal disease in Pima Indians with non-insulin-dependent diabetes mellitus. Diabetic Renal Disease Study Group. *N Engl J Med* 1996; **335**(22): 1636–1642.

Nelson RG, Meyer TW, Myers BD, Bennett PH. Clinical and pathological course of renal disease in non-insulin-dependent diabetes mellitus: the Pima Indian experience. *Semin Nephrol* 1997; **17**(2): 124–131.

Niazy S, Feldt-Rasmussen B, Deckert T. Microalbuminuria in insulin-dependent diabetes: prevalence and practical consequences. *J Diabetes Complications* 1987; **1**(3): 76–80.

Nishimura C, Hotta Y, Gui T, Seko A, Fujimaki T, Ishikawa T, Hayakawa M, Kanai A, Saito T. The level of erythrocyte aldose reductase is associated with the severity of diabetic retinopathy. *Diabetes Res Clin Pract* 1997; **37**(3): 173–177.

Ohkubo Y, Kishikawa H, Araki E, Mitaya T, Isami S, Motoyoshi S, Kojima Y, Furuyoshi N, Shichiri M. Intensive insulin therapy prevents the progression of diabetic microvascular complications in Japanese patients with non-insulin-dependent diabetes mellitus: a randomized, prospective, 6-year study. *Diabetes Res Clin Pract* 1995; **28**(2): 103–117.

Panzram G. Mortality and survival in type 2 (non-insulin-dependent) diabetes mellitus. *Diabetologia* 1987; **30**: 123–131.

Partanen J, Niskanen L, Lehtinen J, Mervaala E, Siitonen O, Uusitupa M. Natural history of peripheral neuropathy in patients with non-insulin-dependent diabetes mellitus. *N Engl J Med* 1995; **333**(2): 89–94.

Parving HH, Tarnow L, Rossing P. Renal protection in diabetes: an emerging role for calcium antagonists. *J Hypertens Suppl* 1996; **14**(4): 21–25.

Perez A, Caixas A, Carreras G, Mauricio D, Pou JM, Serrat J, Gomez-Gerique J, de Leiva A. Lipoprotein compositional abnormalities in type I diabetes: effects of improved glycaemic control. *Diabetes Res Clin Pract* 1997; **36**(2): 83–90.

Ravid M, Brosh D, Ravid-Safran D, Levy Z, Rachmani R.   Main risk factors for nephropathy in type 2 diabetes mellitus are plasma cholesterol levels, mean blood pressure, and hyperglycemia. *Arch Intern Med* 1998; **158**(9): 998–1004.

Ravid M, Lang R, Rachmani R, Lishner M.   Long-term renoprotective effect of angiotensin-converting enzyme inhibition in non-insulin-dependent diabetes mellitus. A 7-year follow-up study. *Arch Intern Med* 1996; **156**(3): 286–289.

Romano G, Patti L, Innelli F, Di Marino L, Annuzzi G, Iavicoli M, Coronel GA, Riccardi G, Rivallese AA. Insulin and sulfonylurea therapy in NIDDM patients. Are the effects on lipoprotein metabolism different even with similar blood glucose control? *Diabetes* 1997; **46**(10): 1601–1606.

Ruggiero-Lopez D, Rellier N, Lecomte M, Lagarde M, Wiernsperger N.   Growth modulation of retinal microvascular cells by early and advanced glycation products. *Diabetes Res Clin Pract* 1997; **34**(3): 135–142.

Salonen JT, Lakka TA, Lakka HM, Valkonen VP, Everson SA, Kaplan GA. Hyperinsulinemia is associated with the incidence of hypertension and dyslipidemia in middle-aged men. *Diabetes* 1998; **47**(2): 270–275.

Sandeman DD, Shore AC, Tooke JE. Relation of kin capillary pressure in patients with insulin-dependent diabetes mellitus to complications and metabolic control. *N Engl J Med* 1992; **327**(11): 760–764.

Sawicki PT. Stabilization of glomerular filtration rate over 2 years in patients with diabetic nephropathy under intensified therapy regimens.   Diabetes Treatment and Teaching Programmes Working Group. *Nephrol Dial Transplant* 1997; **12**(9): 1890–1899.

Selby JV, FitzSimmons SC, Newman JF, Katz PP, Sepe S, Showstack J.   The natural history and epidemiology of diabetic nephropathy. *JAMA* 1990; **263**(14): 1954–1960.

Sima AAF, Bril V, Nathaniel V, McEwan TA, Brown MB, Lattimer SA, Greene DA. Regeneration and repair of myelinated fibers in sural-nerve biopsy specimens from patients with diabetic neuropathy treated with sorbinil. *N Engl J Med* 1988; **319**(9): 548–555.

Skolnick AA. Novel therapies to prevent diabetic retinopathy. *JAMA* 1997; **278**(18): 1480–1481.

Sobenin IA, Tertov VV, Orekhov AN. Atherogenic modified LDL in diabetes. *Diabetes* 1996; **45**(Suppl 3): 35–39.

Takeda H, Yano T, Kishikawa H, Miyata T, Shinohara M, Yamaguchi E, Kobori S, Fan JL, Tokunaga O, Shichiri M. Abnormalities in platelets and vascular endothelial cells induced by glycated lipoproteins. *Intern Med* 1992; **31**(6): 746–751.

Thomas PK.   Classification, differential diagnosis, and staging of diabetic peripheral neuropathy. *Diabetes* 1997; **46**(Suppl 2): 54–57.

Tomlinson DR, Willars GB, Carrington AL. Aldose reductase inhibitors and diabetic complications. *Pharmacol Ther* 1992; **54**(2): 151–194.

Tooke JE. Microvascular function in human diabetes. A physiological perspective. *Diabetes* 1995; **44**(7): 721–726.

UKPDS Group. Intensive blood glucose control with sulphonylureas or insulin compared with conventional treatment and risk of complications in patients with type 2 diabetes (UKPDS 33). *Lancet* 1998; **352**: 837–853.

University Group Diabetes Program. A study of the effects of hypoglycemic agents on vascular complications in patients with adult-onset diabetes. II. Mortality results. *Diabetes* 1970; **19**(Suppl 2): 785–830.

Valensi P, Behar A, Attalah M, Cohen-Boulakia F, Paries J, Attali JR. Increased capillary filtration of albumin in diabetic patients – relation with gender, hypertension, microangiopathy, and neuropathy. *Metabolism* 1998; **47**(5): 503–507.

van Gerven JA, Lemkes HH, van Dijk JG. Long-term effects of tolrestat on symptomatic diabetic sensory polyneuropathy. *J Diabetes Complications* 1992; **6**(1): 45–48.

Wautier JL, Wautier MP, Schmidt AM, Anderson GM, Hori O, Zoukourian C, Capron L, Chappey O, Yan SD, Brett J, et al. Advanced glycation end products (AGEs) on the surface of diabetic erythrocytes bind to the vessel wall via a specific receptor inducing oxidant stress in the vasculature: a link between surface-associated AGEs and diabetic complications. *Proc Natl Acad Sci USA* 1994; **91**(16): 7742–7746.

World Health Organization (WHO). Prevention of diabetes mellitus. In: *WHO Technical Report Series No. 844.* Geneva: WHO, 1994.

Yegin A, Ozben T, Yegin H. Glycation of lipoproteins and accelerated atherosclerosis in non-insulin-dependent diabetes mellitus. *Int J Clin Lab Res* 1995; **25**(3): 157–161.

3

CURRENT TREATMENT STRATEGIES
TO PREVENT DIABETES

A growing understanding of the etiology and pathogenesis of diabetes has strengthened the view that it may be a preventable disease. In addition, the identification of potential risk factors has created the opportunity for early intervention. Principal approaches to the prevention of type 1 diabetes include the regulation of autoimmune responses and protection of β-cells, while diet and exercise remain the cornerstones of preventive therapy for type 2 patients. Considerable interest has also arisen over the role of insulin sensitizing agents in preventing or delaying the onset of type 2 diabetes.

THERAPIES TO PREVENT TYPE 1 DIABETES

Type 1 diabetes is preceded by a period of autoimmunity that can exist for years prior to the onset of symptoms. This pre-diabetic phase is characterized by the presence of particular autoantigens in most patients, including islet cell antibodies (ICA), glutamic acid decarboxylase (GAD) antibodies, insulin autoantibodies (IAA), and tyrosine phosphatase (IA-2) antibodies. While these markers have varying degrees of predictive value for the development of type 1 diabetes, they appear to provide fairly accurate assessments when used in combination (Bingley et al., 1997; Christie et al., 1997). The ability to identify individuals in the pre-diabetic stage provides an opportunity for intervention to prevent the autoimmune destruction of pancreatic cells. Strategies under consideration for the prevention of type 1 diabetes include the induction of immunotolerance and the protection of β-cells from damage.

Induction of Immunotolerance

Autoantigen-Mediated Immunotolerance

Autoantigens such as ICA, GAD, IAA, and IA-2 provide both a basis for the prediction of type 1 diabetes and rational targets for the development of preventive therapies. It has been postulated that the exogenous introduction of autoantigens associated with the development of diabetes may result in immunotolerance and reduced autoimmune damage to pancreatic cells (Ramiya et al., 1996). In support of this approach, several reports have indicated that the intravenous or subcutaneous administration of various islet antigens delays or prevents the onset of diabetes in the non-obese diabetic (NOD) mouse and BioBreeding (BB) rat (Tisch et al., 1994; Ramiya et al., 1997; Daniel & Wegmann, 1996; Kaufman et al., 1993; Gotfredsen et al., 1985). The suppression of immune responses is thought to be T-cell-mediated, due to either clonal anergy and deletion of autoreactive T-cells or the shifting of autoimmune T-helper cell (Th) responses from a destructive (Th1) to a protective (Th2) profile (Figure 3.1).

The induction of tolerance, rather than sensitization, to an exogenous antigen is dependent upon several factors, including the nature of the antigen, its concentration or dose, and the route of administration (Winter et al., 1997). For example, a particular type of tolerance is associated with the introduction of an antigen across a mucous membrane, via inhalation, oral, or nasal administration. Although the mechanism is not clearly understood, it is thought that this type of tolerance may have evolved in order to prevent hypersensitivity to environmental agents (Holt & McMenamin, 1989). The administration of aerosol insulin is associated with the induction of regulatory T-cells (CD8γδ) in NOD mice, which appears to confer immunoprotection and a reduced risk of diabetes (Harrison et al., 1996). Similarly, both intranasal and oral insulin have demonstrated the ability to slow or prevent the development of diabetes in this animal model (Daniel & Wegmann, 1996; Zhang et al., 1991). Oral, nasal, and inhaled antigens may also offer a more convenient mode of preventive therapy than intravenous or subcutaneous delivery in human patients.

Insulin is currently the most extensively studied autoantigen in humans, as it is the only β-cell specific autoantigen associated with diabetes. Initial insulin therapy is associated with partial recovery of β-cell function in many patients, and more intensive insulin administration appears to result in greater improvement. In two small studies of patients newly diagnosed with type 1 diabetes, intensive insulin therapy was associated with

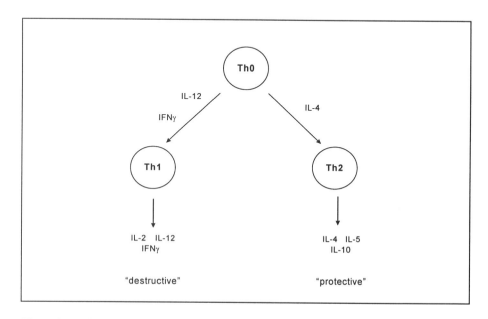

Figure 3.1 - Alternative T-helper response pathways.

improved β-cell function during the subsequent year (Shah et al., 1989), and up to five years later (Linn et al., 1996). However, as changes in immune markers were not evaluated in these studies, the results could be explained by non-immune mechanisms, including β-cell rest and increased insulin sensitivity. A multicenter, randomized, double-blind, controlled trial (IMDIAB VII) is currently underway to determine the efficacy of adding oral insulin to subcutaneous insulin in the protection of residual β-cell function in patients with recent-onset type 1 diabetes (Pozzilli, 1998).

Moreover, a randomized, controlled pilot study (n=14) demonstrated that a combination of intravenous and subcutaneous insulin delayed the onset of overt diabetes in high-risk relatives of patients with type 1 disease (5.0 versus 2.3 years, $p<0.03$; Fuchtenbusch et al., 1998). Two additional, multicenter trials are now being conducted to assess the effects of insulin treatment in non-diabetic, high-risk individuals. The Diabetes Prevention Trial 1 (DPT-1) is designed to determine if insulin treatment can delay or prevent type 1 diabetes in ICA-positive, first-degree relatives (ages 3–45 years) or second- and third-degree relatives (ages less than 20 years) of patients with the disease (Honeyman et al., 1997). In those patients with a projected 5-year risk greater than 50%, insulin is administered intravenously for 1 week per year, and subcutaneously twice daily during the remainder of the year. Patients with a projected 5-year risk of 25–50% receive oral insulin or placebo. In the randomized, double-blind, placebo-controlled European Prediabetes Prevention – SubCutaneous Insulin Trial (EPP-SCIT), pre-diabetic siblings (children and adolescents) at high risk for type 1 diabetes will be evaluated to determine the efficacy of subcutaneous insulin in disease prevention (Coutant et al., 1997). Results of these two trials are expected to be released in 1999 or 2000.

In addition, a double-blind, placebo-controlled, crossover trial of intranasal insulin was conducted in children and young adults with a greater than 50% 5-year risk of developing type 1 diabetes. The one-year study involved the administration of insulin or placebo daily for 10 days, then once-weekly during the remainder of each six-month treatment period. This study was scheduled to be completed at the end of 1998 (Skolnick, 1997).

Non-Specific Immunotolerance

In animal models of diabetes, generalized immune system stimulation has been shown to reduce disease development and progression. This effect has been observed with the administration of various immunomodulators, including complete Freund's adjuvant (CFA) or vaccines such as *bacillus* Calmette-Guérin (BCG). For example, a single injection of CFA was shown to reduce or prevent the development of diabetes in NOD mice and BB rats (Sadelain et al., 1990a, 1990b), and to inhibit autoimmunity and disease recurrence after pancreatic islet transplantation in mice with overt diabetes (Ulaeto et al., 1992). Cell mixing studies indicated that these protective effects may have been due to the generation of splenic non-specific suppressor cells (Qin et al., 1992; McInerney et al., 1991). Other reports have suggested that CFA administration results in a diversion of the autoimmune response from a destructive (Th1) to a non-destructive (Th2) pathway, as the reduced incidence of diabetes with adjuvant administration is associated with decreased interferon γ (IFNγ) and increased interleukin 4 (IL-4) production (Calcinaro et al., 1997; Shehadeh et al., 1993).

Single injections of live BCG have also been shown to inhibit insulitis and the development of overt diabetes in NOD mice. Similar to the results obtained with CFA, splenic cell transfer from vaccinated NOD mice conferred protection against diabetes in the recipient mice, suggesting the involvement of suppressor cells (Harada et al., 1990). Extensive human experience with BCG as a vaccine for tuberculosis makes BCG therapy an attractive candidate for clinical study in diabetes. In a preliminary trial conducted in 17 newly-diagnosed type 1 diabetic patients, a single subcutaneous injection of BCG vaccine led to clinical remission in 65% of patients within four weeks, compared to only 7% of patients in a historical cohort (2 of 29 patients). No adverse effects were reported, and remission was sustained for 6–10 months in 3 of the patients (Shehadeh et al., 1994). However, epidemiological studies have not supported a protective role of BCG vaccination against type 1 diabetes (Parent et al., 1997; Dahlquist & Gothefors, 1995). Moreover, a randomized, double-blind trial (IMDIAB V) comparing BCG vaccination plus nicotinamide with nicotinamide alone in 72 newly diagnosed patients with type 1 diabetes did not find a difference in long-term clinical remission between the two groups (Pozzilli, 1997).

Alternative strategies to induce generalized immunotolerance are the administration of cholera toxin or the diphtheria tetanus toxoid acellular pertussis (DTP) vaccine, alone or conjugated to autoantigen. Both approaches have demonstrated protective effects in NOD mice (Sobel et al., 1998; Bergerot et al., 1997; Ramiya et al., 1996). In addition, various cytokines or cytokine inhibitors may potentially be used to direct the immune response from self-aggression to self-tolerance. However, these approaches will require careful clinical evaluation, as the success of general immunotolerance as a preventive strategy in animal models has not generally been followed by observations of efficacy in humans.

Protection of the β-Cell

As the destruction of pancreatic β-cells appears to be mediated at least in part by the generation of cytokines and free radicals (Rabinovitch et al., 1996; Cunningham & Green, 1994), antioxidant therapy has emerged as a potential strategy to prevent or limit cell death and the development of diabetic symptoms. Nicotinamide (NA), a soluble B-group vitamin, has been shown to protect β-cells from noxious stimuli *in vitro* (Eizirik et al., 1994; Kallman et al., 1992), and has a favorable safety profile in human subjects. An early study conducted in children at high risk for the development of type 1 diabetes supported a protective effect of NA; only 1 of 14 treated children developed the disease, while all 8 of the untreated controls progressed to symptomatic diabetes by the end of the study (Elliot & Chase, 1991). NA treatment was also associated with an improvement in insulin secretion in an open pilot study of individuals with a high risk of type 1 diabetes (Manna et al., 1992).

However, NA treatment at the time of diagnosis does not appear to consistently slow or prevent the progression of the disease, suggesting that its beneficial effects may be dependent upon early intervention and limited existing β-cell damage (Taboga et al., 1994; Lewis et al., 1992; Chase et al., 1990). The patient's age at diagnosis may also be a factor, as the IMDIAB III trial found that NA was more effective than placebo in protecting residual β-cell function only in patients diagnosed after the age of 15 (Pozzilli et al., 1995). Another study indicated that even in at-risk individuals without overt diabetes, NA was ineffective in those for whom metabolic impairment was evident (Herskowitz et al., 1989). Thus, clinical studies of NA therapy have largely focused on prevention in non-diabetic individuals with a high risk of disease development, but normal metabolic function at baseline.

Two multicenter studies have been designed to test the capacity of NA therapy to prevent or slow the onset of type 1 diabetes. The randomized, placebo-controlled Deutsche Nicotinamide Intervention Study (DENIS) evaluated NA therapy or placebo in 55 children (ages 3–12) with a high risk of disease, based on diagnosis in a first-degree relative and high titers of ICA ($\geq$ 20 Juvenile Diabetes Foundation units [JDF]). The trial was terminated after an interim analysis which indicated that NA did not reduce the incidence of diabetes by the targeted rate (from 30% to 6%) at the 3-year timepoint (Lampeter et al., 1998). However, due to the small sample size, this study may not have detected smaller but potentially meaningful reductions in the occurrence of diabetes. In addition, as type 1 diabetes progresses more rapidly in children, these results may not be applicable to an older population (Pozzilli, 1998). The larger, prospective, randomized, double-blind European Nicotinamide Diabetes Intervention Trial (ENDIT) will evaluate the ability of NA to reduce the incidence of type 1 diabetes by 35% or more in ICA-positive ($\geq$ 20 JDF) juvenile, adolescent, and adult first-degree relatives of diagnosed patients. Over 500 subjects, ages 5–40, have entered the 5-year study, which is expected to be completed in 2002 (Pozzilli, 1998).

THERAPIES TO PREVENT TYPE 2 DIABETES

As an unhealthy diet and sedentary lifestyle are well-established risk factors for the development of type 2 diabetes, preventive strategies for this disease have largely focused upon behavioral interventions. Support for this approach was recently reported in the 6-year Da Qing Study (Pan et al., 1997). In this randomized, controlled trial, diet, exercise, and diet-plus-exercise interventions were shown to reduce the risk of diabetes by 31%, 46%, and 42%, respectively, in 577 patients with impaired glucose tolerance. The Oslo Diet and Exercise Study (n=219) also found that a combination of diet and exercise significantly reduced insulin resistance in non-diabetic individuals treated for one year (Torjesen et al., 1997). A similar, randomized, multicenter trial (the Diabetes Prevention Study) is currently underway in Finland to assess the effects of lifestyle intervention in individuals (ages 40–64) with impaired glucose tolerance and a body mass index $\geq$25 (Bloomgarden, 1997).

Potential pharmacological prevention strategies include the use of compounds designed to reduce insulin resistance in individuals at high risk for type 2 diabetes. Such an intervention may inhibit the progression of impaired glucose tolerance and insulin resistance to overt diabetes. For example, the insulin-sensitizing agent troglitazone has demonstrated the ability to improve insulin sensitivity and β-cell responses to glucose in subjects with impaired glucose tolerance (Cavaghan et al., 1997). Troglitazone also appears to improve glucose tolerance and insulin resistance in obese individuals with or without abnormal glucose tolerance (Nolan et al., 1994). Two large trials are currently underway to test the effects of pharmacological strategies in the prevention of type 2 diabetes. The Diabetes Prevention Project (DPP) will assess the efficacy of pharmacotherapy or behavioral modification in nearly 4000 high-risk individuals randomized to one of three groups: 1) metformin, a biguanide which reduces insulin resistance and the production of glucose in the liver; 2) lifestyle changes (7% loss of body weight and an increase in caloric expenditure of at least 700 kcal/week); or 3) placebo (Bloomgarden, 1997). This trial originally included a troglitazone treatment group, but it was discontinued after concerns for liver toxicity increased. In addition, the Troglitazone in the Prevention of Diabetes (TRIPOD) study is designed to evaluate the prophylactic effects of chronic troglitazone administration in women with prior gestational diabetes (Azen et al., 1998). A third study in patients with impaired glucose tolerance is planned, and will evaluate the effects of troglitazone on the progression to type 2 diabetes (Scrip No. 2390, 1998).

CONCLUSIONS

The continuing progress that has been made in understanding the pathogenesis of diabetes has provided a strong rationale for the development of preventive strategies. Numerous approaches have demonstrated promise in animal models of diabetes, and are under active investigation in individuals either at risk for, or in the early stages of, the disease. While initial clinical results with these approaches have been somewhat ambiguous, information from larger, more definitive trials will become available at the beginning of the next century. Whatever the results, the field of diabetes prevention and early intervention is likely to remain a focus of future research.

References

Azen SP, Peters RK, Berkowitz K, Kjos S, Xiang A, Buchanan TA. TRIPOD (Troglitazone In the Prevention Of Diabetes): a randomized, placebo-controlled trial of troglitazone in women with prior gestational diabetes mellitus. *Control Clin Trials* 1998; **19**(2): 217–231.

Bergerot I, Ploix C, Petersen J, Moulin V, Rask C, Fabien N, Lindblad M, Mayer A, Czerkinksky C, Holmgren J, et al. A cholera toxoid-insulin conjugate as an oral vaccine against spontaneous autoimmune diabetes. *Proc Natl Acad Sci USA* 1997; **94**(9): 4610–4614.

Bingley PJ, Bonifacio E, Williams AJ, Genovese S, Bottazzo GF, Gale EA. Prediction of IDDM in the general population: strategies based on combinations of autoantibody markers. *Diabetes* 1997; **46**(11): 1701–1710.

Bloomgarden ZT. Obesity, diabetes prevention, and type 1 diabetes. American Diabetes Association Annual Meeting, 1997. *Diabetes Care* 1997; **20**(12): 1913–1917.

Calcinaro F, Gambelunghe G, Lafferty KJ. Protection from autoimmune diabetes by adjuvant therapy in the non-obese diabetic mouse: the role of interleukin-4 and interleukin-10. *Immunol Cell Biol* 1997; **75**(5): 467–471.

Cavaghan MK, Ehrmann DA, Byrne MM, Polonsky KS. Treatment with the oral antidiabetic agent troglitazone improves beta cell responses to glucose in subjects with impaired glucose tolerance. *J Clin Invest* 1997; **100**(3): 530–537.

Chase HP, Butler-Simon N, Garg S, McDuffie M, Hoops SL, O'Brien D. A trial of nicotinamide in newly diagnosed patients with type 1 (insulin-dependent) diabetes mellitus. *Diabetologia* 1990; **33**(7): 444–446.

Christie MR, Roll U, Payton MA, Hatfield EC, Ziegler AG. Validity of screening for individuals at risk for type I diabetes by combined analysis of antibodies to recombinant proteins. *Diabetes Care* 1997; **20**(6): 965–970.

Coutant R, Carel JC, Timsit J, Boitard C, Bougnères P. Insulin and the prevention of insulin-dependent diabetes mellitus. *Diabete Metab* 1997; **23**(Suppl 3): 25–28.

Cunningham JM, Green IC. Cytokines, nitric oxide, and insulin secreting cells. *Growth Regul* 1994; **4**(4): 173–180.

Dahlquist G, Gothefors L. The cumulative incidence of childhood diabetes mellitus in Sweden unaffected by BCG-vaccination [letter]. *Diabetologia* 1995; **38**(7): 873–874.

Daniel D, Wegmann DR. Protection of nonobese diabetic mice from diabetes by intranasal or subcutaneous administration of insulin peptide B (9-23). *Proc Natl Acad Sci USA* 1996; **93**(2): 956–960.

Eizirik DL, Sandler S, Welsch N, Bendtzen K, Hellerstrom C. Nicotinamide decreases nitric oxide production and partially protects human pancreatic islets against the suppressive effects of combinations of cytokines. *Autoimmunity* 1994; **19**(3): 193–198.

Elliot RB, Chase HP. Prevention or delay of type 1 (insulin-dependent) diabetes mellitus in children using nicotinamide. *Diabetologia* 1991; **34**(5): 362–365.

Fuchtenbusch M, Pabl W, Grassl B, Bachmann W, Standl E, Ziegler AG. Delay of type I diabetes in high risk, first degree relatives by parenteral antigen administration: the Schwabing Insulin Prophylaxis Pilot Trial. *Diabetologia* 1998; **41**(5): 536–541.

Gotfredsen CF, Buschard K, Frandsen EK. Reduction of diabetes incidence of BB Wistar rats by early prophylactic insulin treatment of diabetes-prone animals. *Diabetologia* 1985; **28**: 933–935.

Harada M, Kishimoto Y, Makino S. Prevention of overt diabetes and insulitis in NOD mice by a single BCG vaccination. *Diabetes Res Clin Pract* 1990; **8**(2): 85–89.

Harrison LC, Dampsey-Collier M, Kramer DR, Takahashi K. Aerosol insulin induces regulatory CD8 γδ T cells that prevent murine insulin-dependent diabetes. *J Exp Med* 1996; **184**(6): 2167–2174.

Herskowitz RD, Jackson RA, Soeldner JS, Eisenbarth GS. Pilot trial to prevent Type 1 diabetes: progression to overt IDDM despite oral nicotinamide. *Autoimmunity* 1989; **2**: 733–737.

Holt PG, McMenamin C. Defense against allergic sensitization in the healthy lung: the role of inhalation tolerance. *Clin Exp Allergy* 1989; **19**(3): 255–262.

Honeyman M, Wasserfall C, Nerup J, Rossini A. Prediction and prevention of IDDM. *Diabetologia* 1997; **40**: B58–B61.

Kallman B, Burkart V, Kroncke KD, Kolb-Baclofen V, Kolb H. Toxicity of chemically generated nitric oxide towards pancreatic islet cell can be prevented by nicotinamide. *Life Sci* 1992; **51**: 671–678.

Kaufman DL, Clare-Salzler M, Tian J, Forsthuber T, Ting GS, Robinson P, Atkinson MA, Sercarz EE, Tobin AJ, Lehmann PV. Spontaneous loss of T-cell tolerance to glutamic acid decarboxylase in murine insulin-dependent diabetes. *Nature* 1993; **366**(6450): 69–72.

Lampeter EF, Klinghammer A, Scherbaum WA, Heinze E, Haastert B, Giani G, Kolb H. The Deutsche Nicotinamide Intervention Study: an attempt to prevent type 1 diabetes. DENIS Group. *Diabetes* 1998; **47**(6): 980–984.

Lewis CM, Canafax DM, Sprafka JM, Barbosa JJ. Double-blind randomized trial of nicotinamide in early-onset diabetes. *Diabetes Care* 1992; **15**(1): 121–123.

Linn T, Ortac K, Laube H, Federlin K. Intensive therapy in adult insulin-dependent diabetes mellitus is associated with improved insulin sensitivity and reserve: a randomized, controlled, prospective study over 5 years in newly diagnosed patients. *Metabolism* 1996; **45**(12): 1508–1513.

Manna R, Migliore A, Martin LS, Ferrara E, Ponte E, Marietti G, Scuderi F, Cristiano G, Ghirlanda G, Gambassi G. Nicotinamide treatment in subjects at high risk of developing IDDM improves insulin secretion. *Br J Clin Pract* 1992; **46**(3): 177–179.

McInerney MF, Pek SB, Thomas DW. Prevention of insulitis and diabetes onset by treatment with complete Freund's adjuvant in NOD mice. *Diabetes* 1991; **40**(6): 715–725.

Nolan JJ, Ludvik B, Beersen P, Joyce M, Olefsky J. Improvement in glucose tolerance and insulin resistance in obese subjects treated with troglitazone. *N Engl J Med* 1994; **331**(18): 1188–1193.

Pan XR, Li GW, Hu YH, Wang JX, Yang WY, An ZX, Hu ZX, Lin J, Xiao JZ, Cao HB, et al. Effects of diet and exercise in preventing NIDDM in people with impaired glucose tolerance. The Da Qing IGT and Diabetes Study. *Diabetes Care* 1997; **20**(4): 537–544.

Parent ME, Siemiatycki J, Menzies R, Fritschi L, Colle E. Bacille Calmette-Guérin vaccination and incidence of IDDM in Montreal, Canada. *Diabetes Care* 1997; **20**(5): 767–772.

Pozzilli P. BCG vaccine in insulin-dependent diabetes mellitus. IMDIAB Group [letter]. *Lancet* 1997; **349**(9064): 1520–1521.

Pozzilli P, Visalli N, Signore A, Baroni MG, Buzzetti R, Cavallo MG, Boccuni ML, Fava D, Grognoli C, Andreani D, et al. Double-blind trial of nicotinamide in recent-onset IDDM (the IMDIAB III study). *Diabetologia* 1995; **38**(7): 848–852.

Pozzilli P. Prevention of insulin-dependent diabetes mellitus 1998. *Diabet Metab Rev* 1998; **14**: 69–84.

Qin HY, Suarez WL, Parfrey N, Power RF, Rabinovitch A. Mechanisms of complete Freund's adjuvant protection against diabetes in BB rats: induction of non-specific suppressor cells. *Autoimmunity* 1992; **12**(3): 193–199.

Rabinovitch A, Suarez-Pinzon WL, Strynadka K, Lakey JR, Rajotte RV. Human pancreatic islet beta-cell destruction by cytokines involves oxygen free radicals and aldehyde production. *J Clin Endocrinol Metab* 1996; **91**(9): 3197–3202.

Ramiya VK, Shang X-Z, Pharis PG, Wasserfall CH, Stabler TV, Muir AB, Schatz DA, Maclaren NK. Antigen based therapies to prevent diabetes in NOD mice. *J Autoimmun* 1996; **9**(3): 349–356.

Ramiya VK, Shang X-Z, Wasserfall CH, Maclaren NK. Effect of oral and intravenous insulin and glutamic acid decarboxylase in NOD mice. *Autoimmunity* 1997; **26**(3): 139–151.

Sadelain MW, Qin HY, Lauzon J, Singh B. Prevention of type 1 diabetes in NOD mice by adjuvant immunotherapy. *Diabetes* 1990a; **39**(5): 583–589.

Sadelain MW, Qin HY, Sumoski W, Parfrey N, Singh B, Rabinovitch A. Prevention of diabetes in the BB rat by early immunotherapy using Freund's adjuvant. *J Autoimmun* 1990b; **3**(6): 671–680.

Scrip No. 2390. Troglitazone for diabetes prevention. November 25, 1998; p. 19.

Shah SC, Malone JI, Simpson NE. A randomized trial of intensive insulin therapy in newly diagnosed insulin-dependent diabetes mellitus. *N Engl J Med* 1989; **320**(9): 550–554.

Shehadeh N, Calcinaro F, Bradley BJ, Bruchlim I, Vardi P, Lafferty KJ. Effect of adjuvant therapy on development of diabetes in mouse and man. *Lancet* 1994; **343**(8899): 706–707.

Shehadeh NN, LaRosa F, Lafferty KJ. Altered cytokine activity in adjuvant inhibition of autoimmune diabetes. *J Autoimmun* 1993; **6**(3): 291–300.

Skolnick AA. First type 1 diabetes prevention trials. *JAMA* 1997; **277**(14): 1101–1102.

Sobel DO, Yankelevich B, Goyal D, Nelson D, Mazumder A. The B-subunit of cholera toxin induces immunoregulatory cells and prevents diabetes in the NOD mouse. *Diabetes* 1998; **47**(2): 186–191.

Taboga C, Tonutti L, Noacco C. Residual β-cell activity and insulin requirements in insulin-dependent diabetic patients treated from the beginning with high doses of nicotinamide. A two-year follow-up. *Recent Prog Med* 1994; **85**(11): 513–516.

Tisch R, Yang XD, Liblau RS, McDevitt HO. Administering glutamic acid decarboxylase to NOD mice prevents diabetes. *J Autoimmun* 1994; **7**: 845–850.

Torjesen PA, Birkeland KI, Anderssen SA, Hjermann I, Holme I, Urdal P. Lifestyle changes may reverse development of the insulin resistance syndrome. The Oslo Diet and Exercise Study: a randomized trial. *Diabetes Care* 1997; **20**(1): 26–31.

Ulaeto D, Lacy PE, Kipnis DM, Kanagawa O, Unanue ER. A T-cell dormant state in the autoimmune process of nonobese diabetic mice treated with complete Freund's adjuvant. *Proc Natl Acad Sci USA* 1992; **89**(9): 3927–3931.

Winter WE, House DV, Schatz D. Pharmacological approaches to the prevention of autoimmune diabetes. *Drugs* 1997; **53**(6): 943–956.

Zhang I, Davidson L, Eisenbarth G, Weiner HL. Suppression of diabetes in non-obese diabetic mice by oral administration of porcine insulin. *Proc Natl Acad Sci USA* 1991; **88**: 10252–10256.

4

CURRENT TREATMENT STRATEGIES
TO IMPROVE GLYCEMIC CONTROL

When Banting and Best succeeded in isolating insulin from the pancreas of a dog in the 1920s, it was generally thought that a cure for diabetes had been discovered. However, it soon became clear that although insulin was a major breakthrough in the treatment of diabetes, complications were still inevitable in most patients. In the 1950's, the first oral preparations to treat diabetic patients with residual β-cell function were developed, offering an alternative to insulin in the type 2 population. For decades, attempts have been made to improve upon these therapies, and to design compounds that permit a closer approximation of physiological metabolic control. This challenge has resulted in the development of many novel treatment strategies, and the growth of a stronger and more diverse armamentarium of antidiabetic therapies.

THE BASIS FOR SEEKING EUGLYCEMIA

The primary goal of antidiabetic therapy is the attainment of euglycemia. Obviously, the first objective is to prevent acute metabolic crises (i.e. ketoacidosis, hypoglycemia); however, there is now clear evidence that the improvement of glycemic control also has substantial long-term benefits. The landmark Diabetes Control and Complications Trial (DCCT) demonstrated that intensive glycemic control reduces the development and progression of microvascular complications in patients with type 1 diabetes (DCCT Research Group, 1993). Moreover, subsequent analysis of DCCT results did not identify a glycemic control threshold, indicating that the even small reductions in glycemia may be clinically significant, and that the risk of complications continues to decrease with progressively greater control (DCCT Research Group, 1996). While the benefits of meticulous glycemic control on the development of complications in type 2 diabetes have been debated, the 6-year, prospective Kumamoto study (n=110) reported that intensive insulin treatment delayed the onset and progression of retinopathy, nephropathy, and neuropathy in this population (Ohkubo et al., 1995). These findings were confirmed by the recent completion of the United Kingdom Prospective Diabetes Study (UKPDS), which reported that intensive treatment was associated with a 25% risk reduction in microvascular endpoints in type 2 diabetes, even despite an overall increase in HbA_{1c} in both groups over the course of the study (UKPDS Group, 1998a). Collectively, these studies suggest that the reduction of hyperglycemia has the potential to substantially reduce both morbidity and mortality in patients with diabetes.

NON-PHARMACOLOGICAL TREATMENT OPTIONS

Diet and exercise remain the cornerstones of therapy in diabetes, particularly for type 2 diabetic patients. As obesity and a sedentary lifestyle are well-established risk factors for the development of type 2 diabetes and its complications, interventions targeting a reduction in caloric intake and an increase in physical activity are recommended as a first-line treatment strategy (American Diabetes Association, 1996). Diet and exercise interventions are also indicated as adjunctive therapy to normalize blood glucose levels in patients with type 1 diabetes.

Diet

Dietary fat consumption has been shown to predict the progression of impaired glucose tolerance to type 2 diabetes, after adjustments are made for obesity and measures of glycemic control (Marshall et al., 1994). A high intake of "junk foods" high in fat and low in fiber was also shown to increase the risk of diabetes, while vegetables and grains appeared to confer a protective effect (Gittelsohn et al., 1998). Total dietary fat has also been positively associated with hyperinsulinemia in non-diabetic populations, after controlling for sex, ethnicity, obesity, and physical activity (Marshall et al., 1997). Thus, although a reduction of obesity is an important goal of dietary therapy, diet modification may have the capacity to improve glycemic control independent of its effects on weight reduction.

Several dietary strategies have been evaluated in diabetic patients, including very low calorie diets, reductions in saturated fats, and increases in monounsaturated fats or fiber. Very low calorie diets have been shown to improve body mass index and glycemic control in type 2 patients, even when implemented on an intermittent basis (Williams et al., 1998). In some cases, the level of glycemic control achieved enabled patients to discontinue insulin use for up to one year (Paisey et al., 1998). However, difficulties in compliance may render very low calorie diets impractical for long-term therapy. Diets high in monounsaturated fats have been shown to improve both glycemic control and lipid profiles in type 2 patients, without inducing weight gain (Garg, 1998; Campbell et al., 1994), while both positive and negative results have been reported with low saturated fat/high carbohydrate diets (Howard et al., 1991; Abbott et al., 1989). In some studies, high carbohydrate diets were associated with a worsening of glycemic control and elevated triglyceride levels in diabetic patients (Garg et al., 1994; Garg et al., 1992). These mixed results may be due to differences in the dietary carbohydrate-to-fat ratio, or the level of concurrent fiber intake (Riccardi & Rivellese, 1991). The benefits of dietary fiber are also somewhat equivocal, and appear to be dependent upon the type that is used (Würsch & Pi-Sunyer, 1997; Pick et al., 1996; Bruttomesso et al., 1991). Overall, it appears that most diabetic patients are likely to benefit from a diet with moderately increased levels of monounsaturated fat and reduced levels of saturated fat (American Diabetes Association, 1997). Additionally, in patients requiring insulin, smaller, more frequent meals are generally recommended to reduce the occurrence of hypoglycemia.

Although shown to be initially effective in many patients, diet therapy is associated with a high rate of secondary failure. In the UKPDS, patients with type 2 diabetes randomized to receive diet alone became progressively hyperglycemic over a 10-year period, despite only small increases in body weight (UKPDS Group, 1998a). Reduced glycemic control during dietary therapy may be the result of a lack of compliance over long-term periods, or could be caused by a progressive deterioration of β-cell function in type 2 patients (Levy et al., 1998).

Exercise

Increased physical activity is associated with improved glycemic control in both type 1 and type 2 diabetic patients, irrespective of changes in total body weight (Mosher et al., 1998; Yeater et al., 1990; Schneider et al., 1984). The beneficial effects of exercise on glucose levels appear to be due to enhanced peripheral insulin sensitivity and increased glucose uptake by skeletal muscle (Goodyear & Kahn, 1998; Ishii et al., 1998). Even nonvigorous physical activity has been shown to result in significantly greater insulin sensitivity in obese or nonobese individuals with normal glucose tolerance, or patients with type 1 or type 2 diabetes (Mayer-Davis et al., 1998; Lehmann et al., 1997; Agurs-Collins et al., 1997; Braun et al., 1995). Moreover, physical activity is associated with an improvement in lipid profiles in diabetic patients, suggesting that the risk of atherosclerotic complications may also be reduced with an exercise regimen (Lehmann et al., 1997; Yeater et al., 1990).

In patients with type 1 diabetes and insulin- or sulfonylurea-treated patients with type 2 diabetes, however, special consideration must be given to the risk of hypoglycemia with any exercise intervention. As physical activity enhances the utilization of glucose, patients receiving exogenous insulin should monitor blood glucose levels prior to and after exercising, in order to identify when changes in insulin or food intake may be necessary. Blood glucose responses to prolonged physical activity have been shown to be consistent in type 1 patients when pre-exercise meals and insulin regimen are kept constant, suggesting that hypoglycemia may be avoided with the use of a regular routine (Temple et al., 1995).

INSULIN

Insulin therapy is indicated in all patients with type 1 diabetes, as well as many type 2 patients who are poorly controlled by diet, exercise, and/or oral hypoglycemic agents. Optimal insulin therapy is that which most closely approximates the natural pattern of insulin secretion in non-diabetic individuals; however, this profile has proven difficult to achieve. A breakthrough in insulin therapy occurred with the introduction of semi-synthetic insulins and synthetic human insulins produced by recombinant DNA technology. These insulin products have largely solved the problem of immunogenicity associated with animal insulin preparations (Schernthaner, 1993). More recently, this technology has been used to create insulin analogs with altered pharmacokinetic profiles, designed to provide targeted pharmacodynamic actions.

Insulin can be formulated as short- or rapid-acting (regular), intermediate (NPH, lente) or long-acting (ultralente) preparations. In an attempt to mimic the physiological profile of insulin, a short-acting insulin, taken prior to meals to control postprandial glucose elevations, is often used in combination with an intermediate or long-acting preparation, which provides basal insulin concentrations. However, this strategy often fails to achieve the desired pattern of insulin secretion and glycemic control. Subcutaneous injections of regular insulin require approximately two hours to achieve peak concentrations; thus, doses must be administered at least one half hour prior to meals in order to control postprandial glucose levels (Lean et al., 1985). The need to carefully time meals, coupled with the danger of severe hypoglycemia if a meal is not consumed within a certain time period after the insulin injection, represent significant limitations of this regimen. Moreover, the activity of subcutaneous regular insulin lasts for several hours, which could lead to postprandial hyperinsulinemia and hypoglycemia (Olsson et al., 1988). The occurrence of such events is unpredictable, since insulin by this route has demonstrated high intra-individual variability in pharmacokinetic and pharmacodynamic responses. Finally, conventional intermediate and long-acting insulin formulations injected once daily generally fail to provide adequate basal insulin levels over a 24-h period (Binder et al., 1984).

To improve the action of insulin, "designer" analogs have been developed which include strategic structural alterations. Both rapid-acting and long-acting insulin analogs have thereby been created in attempts to more closely mimic the pattern of natural insulin secretion. The main objective in the development of rapid-acting insulin analogs is to achieve a faster time to peak concentration, combined with a faster return to basal levels. Such a compound could be injected immediately before a meal, offering greater convenience, and possibly a reduced risk of postprandial hypoglycemia.

Rapid-Acting Insulin Analogs: Insulin Lispro

As the slow absorption and metabolism of regular insulin is largely due to its self-association into hexamers in solution (Kang et al., 1991a), attempts have been made to develop insulin analogs with reduced self-association through the introduction of charge repulsion, stearic manipulations, or removal of metal-binding sites (Barnett and Owens, 1997). Monomeric and dimeric insulin analogs have demonstrated a rapid onset of action, with good postprandial glycemic control following administration immediately prior to meals (Kang et al., 1991b; Nielsen et al., 1995). However, the structural alterations that increase the diffusion capabilities of some insulin analogs have also led to some untoward effects. For example, one analog (Asp^{B10}) was found to possess carcinogenic properties in rats, potentially due to an increased affinity for insulin-like growth factor I receptors (Drejer, 1992; Bornfeldt et al., 1991); the development of this compound was consequently discontinued.

Insulin lispro (Humalog,® Eli Lilly and Co.), which was approved for clinical use in the United States and Europe in 1996, is based on a reversal of the natural sequence of proline at position B28 and lysine at position B29 (Lys^{B28}, Pro^{B29} human insulin). The resulting conformational change stearically hinders the ability of insulin monomers to form dimers in solution (Holleman and Hoekstra, 1997). Clinical trials have confirmed a more rapid onset and offset of action with insulin lispro in comparison to regular insulin, accompanied by improved postprandial blood glucose control in diabetic patients (Torlone et al., 1994). In a randomized, open-label, multicenter, crossover study conducted in 1008 patients with type 1 diabetes (Anderson et al., 1997a), insulin lispro administered immediately prior to meals resulted in significantly lower elevations in postprandial glucose levels than regular human insulin injected 30–45 min prior to meals (50% and 125% lower at the 1h and 2h timepoints, respectively). Similar results were reported in a 6-month study of comparable design conducted in 722 patients with type 2 diabetes. In this study, postprandial elevations in serum glucose levels were 30% lower at 1h and 53% lower at 2h with insulin lispro treatment than with regular human insulin (Anderson et al., 1997b). The improved postprandial performance seen in the insulin lispro-treated patients could be explained in part by sub-optimal timing of the human insulin injections. Indeed, overall glycemic control, as reflected by glycated hemoglobin (HbA_{1c}) levels, did not differ between the two treatment groups.

The reduced self-association of insulin lispro also contributes to a shorter duration of action and a more rapid return to basal levels, which could reduce the occurrence of postprandial hypoglycemia. Several studies in diabetic patients have reported a reduced risk of hypoglycemia with insulin lispro relative to regular human insulin (Anderson et al., 1997a; Anderson et al., 1997b; Holleman et al., 1997; Pfutzner et al., 1996), although others have not reported a difference in incidence between the two treatment regimens (Vignati et al., 1997; Daniels et al., 1997). Collectively, these studies suggest that insulin lispro may improve postprandial glucose control without increasing the risk of hyperinsulinemia or hypoglycemia in patients with type 1 and type 2 diabetes. In addition, the enhanced convenience of immediate injection before meals is likely responsible for the greater health-related quality of life ratings reported for insulin lispro in comparison to regular insulin (Kostanos et al., 1997).

As mentioned above, insulin lispro has not been shown to improve overall glycemic control in diabetic patients, as measured by fasting glucose or HbA_{1c} (Davey et al., 1997). This finding is not surprising, since HbA_{1c} is more dependent upon basal insulin control. Studies are currently underway to optimize the combination of insulin lispro with prolonged-action basal insulin therapy (Campbell et al., 1996). Although most clinical trials have included NPH or ultralente as basal insulin therapy, other candidates are in development, including an intermediate-acting neutral protamine lispro (NPL; Janssen et al., 1997). In addition, recent evidence suggests that insulin lispro may have advantages over regular insulin therapy in reducing HbA_{1c} values when administered as a continuous subcutaneous insulin infusion (Melki et al., 1998; Zinman et al., 1997). However, further study will be necessary to confirm these findings.

Long-Acting Insulin Analogs

A constant, low-level, basal supply of insulin is a necessary component of good glycemic control. Thus, various strategies have been employed to create a long-acting insulin analog capable of maintaining an appropriate and reproducible level of insulin over a 24-h period. However, development in this area has been difficult. An initial long-acting insulin analog, NovoSol Basal, demonstrated prolonged activity in comparison to ultralente insulin due to its crystallization properties *in vivo* (Jorgensen et al., 1989); however, macrophage responses at the site of injection led to discontinuation of its development.

Alternative strategies to produce a long-acting insulin analog include improving the stability of the molecule, increasing the isoelectric point of human insulin to a neutral pH, and binding fatty-acid-acylated insulins to albumin (Barnett & Owens, 1997). HOE 901 (Gly^{A21} di-arginyl^{B30} human insulin), an insulin analog for which major clinical studies have been completed, has demonstrated improved stability and a shift in the isoelectric point to a neutral pH. In healthy volunteers, subcutaneous administration of HOE 901 resulted in a consistent and prolonged plasma insulin profile (Coates et al., 1995a). Despite this prolonged duration of action, HOE 901 does not appear to promote mitogenesis *in vitro* as was the case for the Asp^{B10} analog (Berti et al., 1998). In addition, human insulin acylated with fatty acids at Lys B29 and bound to serum albumin has demonstrated protracted activity in an animal model of diabetes (Myers et al., 1997), without reports of injection-site inflammatory reactions (Markussen et al., 1996). Compounds such as these may provide longer-lasting basal insulin levels, and profiles which more closely mimic normal physiological insulin secretion.

Insulin Delivery Systems

Although significant advances have been made in the development of insulin formulations that more closely mimic normal endogenous insulin secretion, new delivery techniques are necessary to optimize the use of these therapies. Currently, subcutaneous injection is the predominant mode of insulin delivery, and has recently been improved with the development of "pen" injectors that enhance accuracy and convenience (Graff & McClanahan, 1998). However, the shortcomings of this method include slow absorption and elimination, lack of a portal-peripheral insulin gradient, failure to achieve optimal basal insulin levels, and a high risk of hypoglycemia with intensive therapy. Intravenous delivery provides a more physiologically accurate pattern of postprandial insulin levels, with rapid peaking and elimination; however, this method is untenable for long-term therapy. Thus, several alternative delivery techniques are currently under investigation, in order to improve both the effectiveness and convenience of insulin therapy.

Continuous Infusion (Insulin Pumps)

Continuous subcutaneous insulin infusion (CSII), achieved with the use of external pumps, has been developed as a potential means of maintaining adequate basal insulin levels. In type 1 diabetic patients, CSII is associated with a reduced incidence of hypoglycemia in comparison to multiple injections, with no adverse effects on glycemic control (Kanc et al., 1998; Bode et al., 1996). However, due to the slow absorption of subcutaneously administered insulin, levels are not easily adjusted to meet patient needs at any given time. In addition, the use of conventional insulin with this system cannot adequately provide acute delivery of a meal-related bolus (Hoffman & Ziv, 1997). Evaluations of glycemic control in patients with type 1 diabetes have not generally supported an advantage of this type of therapy over multiple subcutaneous injections (Marshall et al., 1987; Schiffrin & Belmonte, 1982), although differences favoring CSII have been reported in patients with type 2 disease (Jennings et al., 1991).

Improved absorption of pump-delivered insulin may be possible with intraperitoneal, rather than subcutaneous, administration. Intraperitoneal insulin, delivered via an implantable pump with external remote control, is preferentially absorbed into the portal system and delivered to the liver, resulting in a portal-peripheral insulin gradient. This property may reduce the risk of peripheral hyperinsulinemia, a potential risk factor for atherosclerosis. Moreover, intraperitoneal insulin appears to be absorbed more rapidly than subcutaneous insulin injections (Kelley et al., 1996). Clinical trials have demonstrated that continuous intraperitoneal insulin infusion (CIPII) results in more rapid and consistent insulin absorption than CSII in patients with both type 1 and type 2 diabetes (Hermans et al., 1995;

Wredling et al., 1991). Although preliminary studies in type 1 and type 2 diabetic patients indicate that glycemic control is comparable for CIPII, CSII, and conventional insulin therapy, CIPII is associated with the lowest risk of hypoglycemia among these delivery systems (Dunn et al., 1997; Saudek et al., 1996; Olsen et al., 1993). Potential limitations of continuous insulin delivery include the risk of pump and catheter occlusions (Renard et al., 1995). Overall, the reduced risk of hypoglycemia, while achieving comparable metabolic control, represents a possible advantage of continuous insulin delivery over conventional therapy.

Oral Delivery

Oral insulin would clearly offer a more convenient and less invasive treatment option than parenteral therapy. However, the absorption and distribution of orally administered insulin is hindered by factors including proteolysis in the stomach and small intestine, as well as intestinal epithelial cells that prevent macromoleculer transport (Hoffman & Ziv, 1997). Strategies to overcome these barriers include the administration of coated capsules (Gwinup et al., 1991) or insulin-containing nanospheres (Damage et al., 1997), inhibitory agents to reduce enzymolysis (Bernkop-Schnurch, 1998), and/or absorption promoters (Saffran et al., 1991; Ziv et al., 1994). Several of these approaches are in the preliminary stages of development at this time.

Intrapulmonary Delivery

The large surface area and extensive vascularization of the lungs represent two potential advantages of intrapulmonary insulin delivery. In initial studies in healthy volunteers, inhaled insulin resulted in significant elevations of serum insulin, accompanied by reductions in blood glucose (Jendle & Karlberg, 1996a). Moreover, both the onset of action and time to reach maximal metabolic response were more rapid with inhaled insulin than with subcutaneous injections in this healthy population (Heinemann et al., 1997). Significant reductions in plasma fasting glucose have also been observed following the administration of inhaled insulin to patients with type 2 diabetes (Jendle & Karlberg, 1996b; Laube et al., 1993). In all of these studies, intrapulmonary insulin was safe and well tolerated.

However, one potential difficulty with inhaled insulin is its low bioavailability in comparison to injected insulin (Heinemann et al., 1997). To address this problem, the use of large porous particles or absorption enhancers has been suggested as a potential means of increasing bioavailability *in vivo* (Edwards et al., 1997; Yamamoto et al., 1994). In addition, as current inhalers are capable of delivering only a small fraction of drug from the device into the deep lung, novel inhaler devices and insulin formulations are currently under investigation (Service, 1997). For example, a pulmonary delivery system under joint development by Pfizer and Inhale Therapeutics is designed to administer a dry aerosol powder into the deep lung (Scrip No. 2279, 1997). Phase II results with this system have shown that the inhaled insulin resulted in equivalent glycemic control to injected insulin in type 1 and type 2 diabetic patients over a 3-month period (Scrip No. 2345, 1998). In addition, the AERx system being tested by Aradigm and Novo Nordisk is an electronic inhaler which guides the patient's breathing and automatically delivers a precise dose of aerosolized insulin into the lungs (Saudek, 1997). A third method, utilizing a powder form of insulin, is under development by Eli Lilly and Dura Pharmaceuticals (Service, 1997).

Intranasal Delivery

Intranasal delivery is another potential option for convenient and noninvasive insulin therapy. Intranasal insulin is more rapidly absorbed and eliminated than subcutaneous insulin, and appears to be associated with less inter-subject pharmacokinetic variability (Drejer et al., 1992). In addition, local tolerability is favorable with this mode of administration (Coates et al., 1995b; Drejer et al., 1992). However, bioavailability in humans is low, even with the addition of various absorption enhancers (Valensi et al., 1996; Jacobs et al., 1993; Drejer et al., 1992), which will most likely hinder its clinical use. In clinical trials of type 1 and type 2 diabetic patients, mealtime doses of intranasal insulin in combination with intermediate or long-acting conventional insulin therapy failed to improve blood glucose excursions or overall glycemic control (Hilsted et al., 1995; Bruce et al., 1991; Frauman et al., 1987). Thus, due to low absolute bioavailability and a high incidence of treatment failure, intranasal insulin is not a satisfactory alternative to parenteral therapy at this time.

Other Forms of Delivery

Several other modes of insulin delivery have been investigated, including buccal (al-Achi & Greenwood, 1993; Oh & Ritschel, 1990), rectal (Nishihata et al., 1989), colonic (Cheng et al., 1994), ocular (Bartlett et al., 1994) and transdermal administration (Tachibana & Tachibana, 1991). However, these approaches are similarly limited by low insulin bioavailability (Hoffman & Ziv, 1997; Aungst et al., 1988). Further innovations, perhaps in the form of novel formulations, will be necessary before any of these delivery systems can be considered a reasonable alternative to conventional insulin therapy.

PHARMACEUTICAL TREATMENT OPTIONS

Although diet and exercise are always indicated in the treatment of diabetes, most type 2 patients will eventually require the use of oral anti-hyperglycemic agents. The pharmaceutical options for patients with type 2 diabetes have grown substantially over the past few decades with the development of novel strategies to improve glycemic control. Several oral agents have demonstrated efficacy as first-line monotherapy, and may also be used in combination to achieve additional metabolic improvement. In addition, although all patients with type 1 diabetes require insulin therapy, there is some indication that adjunctive use of certain anti-hyperglycemic agents may further improve glycemic control in this population (Hollander et al., 1997; Serrano-Rios et al., 1988).

Sulfonylureas

Sulfonylureas, which have been available since the 1950's, remain a prevalent choice for first-line oral anti-hyperglycemic therapy. Sulfonylureas stimulate insulin secretion by binding to receptors on the β-cell that close potassium channels, resulting in depolarization,

Table 4.1 - Currently available sulfonylurea compounds

First generation compounds:	Newer Generation Compounds
acetohexamide tolazamide tolbutamide chlorpropamide	glibenclamide (glyburide) glipizide glimepiride

an influx of calcium, and the release of insulin (Melander et al., 1989). Reductions in insulin resistance have also been reported with sulfonylurea therapy, but are likely a secondary effect of the enhanced insulin secretion (Greenfield et al., 1982). In patients responding to sulfonylurea therapy, 1–2.6% reductions in HbA_{1c} levels have been reported (UKPDS Group, 1998b; Draeger, 1995). However, it has been estimated that only 60%–70% of patients achieve "good" glycemic control with sulfonylurea therapy, and the majority of severely obese patients do not derive benefit from these compounds (Scheen & Lefebvre, 1998). In addition, sulfonylureas are associated with an increasing rate of secondary failure over time (60% over 6 years; UKPDS Group, 1998b), potentially due to a progressive deterioration of β-cell function.

Hypoglycemia is the most common adverse event associated with the use of sulfonylurea therapy (van Staa et al., 1997), and can be particularly prevalent in elderly patients. Sulfonylurea-induced severe hypoglycemia has been estimated to have a fatality rate of about 10% (Gerich, 1989). Weight gain is common in sulfonylurea-treated patients, and is a significant drawback to therapy in obese individuals (Scheen & Lefebvre, 1998). However, both hypoglycemia and weight gain appear to be less frequent in patients treated with sulfonylureas than in those treated with insulin (UKPDS Group, 1998a). Some have contended that sulfonylurea therapy may contribute to cardiovascular morbidity and mortality by inhibiting potassium-channel-mediated cardioprotective mechanisms, but this issue is still under debate (Brady & Terzic, 1998; Cleveland et al., 1997; Meinert et al., 1970; University Group Diabetes Program, 1970).

Numerous sulfonylureas are currently available for the treatment of diabetes (Table 4.1). Although some reports have indicated that efficacy is comparable for the various compounds (Langtry & Balfour, 1998; Prendergast, 1984), the UKPDS reported that significantly lower HbA_{1c} levels were achieved with chlorpropamide than with glibenclamide (UKPDS Group, 1998a). However, the greater reductions observed with chlorpropamide were accompanied by a higher incidence of hypertension, and did not translate into a lower occurrence of microvascular complications. Overall, some of the newer generation agents (e.g., glipizide and glimepiride) appear to have more favorable safety profiles than older agents (Shorr et al., 1996). In addition, both glipizide and glimepiride are available in once-daily formulations, which may enhance patient compliance.

Biguanides

Biguanide agents reduce hepatic glucose production and improve peripheral insulin sensitivity, enhancing glucose uptake and oxidative metabolism in muscular and adipose tissues. Thus, biguanides target the root of type 2 diabetes pathophysiology, namely, insulin resistance. In addition, biguanides may reduce gastrointestinal glucose absorption, further contributing to an attenuation of hyperglycemia (Bailey, 1992). Metformin, the principal member of this drug class, has demonstrated comparable effects on overall glycemic control to sulfonylurea monotherapy in patients with type 2 diabetes (UKPDS Group, 1998c; Melchior & Jaber, 1996), although metformin appears to be more effective in controlling postprandial hyperglycemia (Melchior & Jaber, 1996). Rates of primary and secondary failure are also similar for metformin and sulfonylurea monotherapy (UKPDS Group, 1998b).

In contrast to sulfonylurea therapy, metformin is not associated with weight gain, and may even contribute to weight loss in some patients (Davidson & Peters, 1997). In addition, metformin may improve lipid profiles, including a reduction in triglyceride levels (Palumbo, 1998; Hollenbeck et al., 1991). These effects suggest that biguanide therapy may be particularly indicated in obese or hyperlipidemic type 2 patients. This view is supported by a recent subanalysis of the UKPDS, which indicated that metformin therapy reduced diabetic complications and death in obese patients to a significantly greater extent than sulfonylurea or insulin therapy (UKPDS Group, 1998c).

The most common adverse events observed with metformin are gastrointestinal effects such as nausea, bloating, diarrhea, and abdominal cramps. These events are generally ameliorated by the concomitant administration of food, and tend to decrease in incidence over time. Hypoglycemic episodes are less prevalent with biguanide therapy than with insulin or sulfonylurea therapy (UKPDS Group, 1998b). The most serious potential side effect of the biguanides is the development of lactic acidosis; this complication led to the removal of the biguanide, phenformin, from clinical use in 1977 (Califano, 1977). However, lactic acidosis occurs more rarely with metformin, and usually in patients with known contraindications to biguanide therapy, such as impaired renal or hepatic function (Wilholm & Myrhed, 1993).

α-Glucosidase Inhibitors

α-Glucosidase inhibitors suppress the activity of α-glucosidase enzymes released in the small intestine. These enzymes are responsible for the hydrolysis of complex carbohydrates into simple sugars. Enzyme inhibition thereby delays simple sugar absorption and reduces postprandial glucose levels. Two currently approved members of this class, acarbose and miglitol, have demonstrated efficacy not only in smoothing postprandial glucose peaks, but also in improving overall metabolic control (Coniff et al., 1995a; Chiasson et al., 1994; Johnston et al., 1994). α-glucosidase inhibitors are associated with improvements in postprandial glucose concentrations that are greater than those observed with sulfonylureas, and similar to metformin (Inoue et al., 1997; Hoffman & Spengler, 1997). However, mean reductions in HbA_{1c} observed with α-glucosidase inhibitors (approximately 0.7%) are smaller than those reported for sulfonylurea or biguanide therapy (Coniff et al., 1995b).

The primary adverse events associated with α-glucosidase inhibitor therapy are flatulence, soft stools, diarrhea, and mild abdominal pain. These effects are due to the bacterial fermentation of undigested carbohydrates in the intestine (Santeusanio & Compagnucci, 1994). Although these symptoms are dose-related and generally diminish with continued use, they may limit initial compliance with therapy. Initiation of therapy with low doses and slow titration may improve tolerability. α-glucosidase inhibitor monotherapy is not associated with hypoglycemia, hyperinsulinemia, or weight gain. However, additive effects in combination therapy with another antidiabetic agent may result in an increased hypoglycemic risk. Though these α-glucosidase inhibitors are not systemically active, metabolites of the compounds are absorbed. Hepatitis associated with acarbose therapy has been reported primarily in Japanese patients who were exposed to relatively high doses when adjusted for body weight. Overall, with appropriate dosing, α-glucosidase inhibitors are safe and effective as combination therapy in patients inadequately controlled by insulin or sulfonylureas alone (Coniff et al., 1995c; Vannasaeng et al., 1995). Moreover, α-glucosidase inhibitors may provide a useful adjunct to insulin therapy in the control of postprandial glucose surges in type 1 diabetic patients (Rios, 1994).

Thiazolidinediones

The thiazolidinediones represent a relatively new class of anti-hyperglycemic agents. Although their mechanism of action has not been fully elucidated, they are primarily characterized as "insulin sensitizers," compounds that enhance the activity of insulin in peripheral tissues. In addition, thiazolidinediones have a small effect in inhibiting hepatic glucose production (Johnson et al., 1998), and may improve β-cell responsiveness to glucose (Prigeon et al., 1998; Cavaghan et al., 1997). However, they are not insulin secretagogues, and thus are not effective in the absence of insulin. The thiazolidinediones have a high affinity for the peroxisome proliferator activator-γ receptor, or PPAR-γ, which regulates the expression of genes encoding for proteins involved in glucose and lipid metabolism (Henry, 1997; Lambe & Tugwood, 1996).

Troglitazone was the first thiazolidinedione to be approved for clinical use in diabetic patients in the U.S. Improvements in fasting and postprandial blood glucose, glucose tolerance, and hyperinsulinemia have been documented with troglitazone therapy in type 2 diabetic patients (Maggs et al., 1998; Suter et al., 1992; Iwamoto et al., 1991) as well as individuals with impaired glucose tolerance (Antonucci et al., 1997; Berkowitz et al., 1996). Some studies have found beneficial effects of troglitazone on lipid profiles (Maggs et al., 1998; Kumar et al., 1996), although this effect has not been consistently reported (Sironi et al., 1997). Other thiazolidinediones in development, such as rosiglitazone and pioglitazone, have demonstrated similar effects on metabolic control (Yamasaki et al., 1997; Clinical Investigator News, 1998). Troglitazone has been associated with only moderate reductions in HbA_{1c} levels (0.5–0.7%) in most studies of the compound as stand-alone therapy (Iwamoto et al., 1996; Iwamoto et al., 1991). Troglitazone is much more effective in patients who are poorly controlled on insulin therapy; average HbA_{1c} levels in troglitazone-treated patients differed from placebo-treated patients by 1.4% in a large, phase III trial (Schwartz et al., 1998). In addition, many troglitazone-treated patients were able to reduce or discontinue insulin therapy.

Although the development of earlier thiazolidinediones (e.g., ciglitazone and englitazone), was discontinued due to toxicity (Scheen, 1997), troglitazone has demonstrated a favorable tolerability profile in clinical studies. The incidence of adverse events with troglitazone therapy was generally similar to that observed with placebo, although a mild reduction in hemoglobin or neutrophil counts has been reported in some patients (Johnson et al., 1998; Kumar et al., 1996). Weight gain is also common. Both hemoglobin and weight findings are due to the drug's effect on fluid distribution among body compartments. The mechanism of this effect has not been determined. Liver dysfunction has also been documented in a small percentage of patients receiving troglitazone, prompting regulatory recommendations for regular hepatic monitoring (Johnson et al., 1998). Despite animal data showing that thiazolidinediones cause heart enlargement and fluid accumulation in the pericardial, pleural, and peritoneal spaces at high doses, no evidence of adverse cardiac effects was found in humans monitored with echocardiography (Ghazzi et al., 1997). In fact, troglitazone may have a beneficial effect on cardiovascular risk factors, as it appears to lower blood pressure and reduce atherosclerosis in both hypertensive and non-hypertensive individuals, potentially due to a reduction of insulin resistance (Minamikawa et al., 1998; Ogihara et al., 1995; Nolan et al., 1994).

Meglitinides

Like the sulfonylureas, meglitinide derivatives stimulate insulin secretion from pancreatic β-cells through the regulation of ATP-sensitive potassium channels. However, the meglitinides are characterized as *nonsulfonylurea* insulin secretagogues, as their activity is mediated by receptors distinct from those affected by sulfonylurea compounds (Fuhlendorff et al., 1998). As these compounds are rapidly absorbed and eliminated, they target the control of postprandial glucose levels (Balfour & Faulds, 1998; Bakkali-Nadi et al., 1994). In this sense, the pharmacodynamic effect of meglitinide therapy is to simulate the physiologic secretion of insulin in response to meals. Thus, meglitinide therapy entails dosing before each meal. While the need to take this drug three or more times a day can be seen as a disadvantage, it also provides much greater dosing flexibility than the long-acting sulfonylureas. The latter therapy requires that meals be eaten throughout the day once the sulfonylurea has been taken in the morning. Meglitinide therapy allows patients to eat on a variable schedule. If a meal and its pre-meal dose are missed, there is less danger of subsequent hypoglycemia.

Several meglitinide compounds are in clinical development, and one (repaglinide) was recently approved for use in type 2 diabetic patients. Improvements in both fasting and postprandial blood glucose have been reported with repaglinide therapy (Wolffenbuttel et al., 1993), and similar effects have been documented with other meglitinides, including A4166 and BTS 67,582 (Kikuchi, 1996; Skillman & Raskin, 1997). Small reductions in fructosamine and HbA_{1c} were also reported for BTS 67,582 in one study (Skillman & Raskin, 1997). Clinical evidence suggests that the meglitinides are comparable to the sulfonylureas in controlling blood glucose levels (Wolffenbuttel et al., 1993).

Due their short duration of action, the meglitinides are associated with a low risk of hypoglycemia (Balfour & Faulds, 1998). In addition, meglitinide derivatives are metabolized in the liver and excreted primarily in the bile, and thus may have an advantage in patients with renal dysfunction (Scheen, 1997). Clinical studies are currently underway to assess the safety and efficacy of meglitinide compounds in combination with other antidiabetic therapies.

Hormonal Strategies

A number of endogenous hormones, in addition to insulin, are involved in the maintenance of normal metabolic function. However, the potential therapeutic value of these hormones in patients with diabetes has only recently been recognized. Two peptide hormones, amylin and glucagon-like peptide 1 (GLP-1), have demonstrated promising anti-hyperglycemic activity in animal models of diabetes and preliminary trials in humans, and could represent a new option for improving metabolic control.

Amylin, or islet amyloid polypeptide, is a peptide hormone that is co-secreted with insulin from pancreatic β-cells. The administration of amylin or its analog has been shown to slow the rate of gastric emptying in diabetic animals and humans, potentially by regulating parasympathetic input to the stomach (Macdonald, 1997). Amylin is altered by a similar extent to insulin in patients with type 1 and 2 diabetes, and in non-diabetic individuals with impaired glucose tolerance (Scherbaum, 1998), suggesting that replacement therapy may help to improve glycemic regulation in these populations.

A synthetic analog of amylin, pramlintide, is currently under development for use in both type 1 and type 2 diabetes. In clinical studies, the subcutaneous administration of pramlintide was associated with a reduction in fasting and postprandial glucose levels, as well as fructosamine, in patients with type 1 diabetes (Thompson et al., 1997a; 1997b). In patients with type 2 diabetes receiving pramlintide in addition to insulin therapy, improvements in fructosamine and cholesterol, accompanied by modest reductions in HbA$_{1c}$ (approximately 0.5%), were also reported (Thompson et al., 1998).

Upper gastrointestinal adverse events, predominantly nausea, appear to be the most common side effects associated with amylin analog therapy (Thompson et al., 1997a; 1997b). These effects are transient, and tend to subside with continued therapy. The incidence of hypoglycemia with pramlintide administration did not differ significantly from placebo in clinical studies. Unlike other anti-hyperglycemic agents, however, pramlintide requires subcutaneous injection up to three or four times daily (at mealtimes), which may limit patient convenience and compliance.

A second peptide under investigation for its therapeutic value in diabetes is GLP-1, a gut hormone that is released into the bloodstream following meals. Although its primary function is to enhance the insulinotropic action of glucose and stimulate insulin secretion from pancreatic β-cells (Shen et al., 1998), GLP-1 has also been shown to inhibit the production of glucagon and to delay gastric emptying (Wishart et al., 1998; Naslund et al., 1998). These effects appear to independently contribute to the inhibition of postprandial glucose levels by GLP-1 in patients with type 2 diabetes (Schirra et al., 1998). In addition to its beneficial effects on postprandial glycemic excursions, the subcutaneous administration of GLP-1 has also resulted in improvements in fasting blood glucose levels in type 2 diabetic patients (Nauck et al., 1998a, 1998b). Finally, GLP-1 appears to promote satiety and to inhibit food intake, which could be a favorable effect in obese diabetic patients (Flint et al., 1998).

As the insulinotropic effect of GLP-1 is dependent upon the presence of normal or high levels of glucose, it has a very low risk of hypoglycemia (Qualmann et al., 1995; Nauck et al., 1993; Nathan et al., 1992). This property may represent an advantage of GLP-1 over currently available therapies. Although GLP-1 requires subcutaneous administration, which could limit patient convenience, the development of orally active analogs is under investigation.

Bromocriptine

Bromocriptine is a dopaminergic agonist that is used to treat acromegaly, a condition frequently associated with glucose intolerance and diabetes, as well as Parkinson's disease and prolactin-secreting pituitary tumors. It has previously been demonstrated that bromocriptine therapy improves glucose tolerance and insulin levels in patients with acromegaly, potentially as a result of its regulatory effects on hormone metabolism (Dolecek et al., 1982; Wang et al., 1979).   Some evidence has accumulated that bromocriptine may have protective effects on pancreatic β-cells in autoimmune-mediated diabetes (Liang et al., 1998; Hawkins et al., 1994). However, clinical studies have not generally supported a significant benefit of bromocriptine in the treatment of type 1 diabetic patients (Atkinson et al., 1990; Scobie et al., 1983).

Animal models suggest that bromocriptine therapy influences carbohydrate and lipid metabolism through a neuroendocrine mechanism (Cincotta et al., 1989).   Central dopaminergic tone appears to be involved in the transition from fuel-storing to fuel-utilizing states in hibernating animals or animals with seasonal circadian rhythms (Cincotta et al., 1993, 1991). Some data suggest that individuals who are obese, diabetic, or both have relatively elevated prolactin levels and, presumably, relatively low central dopaminergic tone (Rojdmark & Rossner, 1991; Mooradian et al., 1985). Bromocriptine therapy is therefore proposed to improve glycemic control and reduce insulin resistance by normalizing this neuroendocrine perturbation (Meier et al., 1992).

In small, uncontrolled clinical studies in type 2 diabetic patients, bromocriptine has been shown to reduce body fat and hyperglycemia (Meier et al., 1992; Barnett et al., 1980). More recently, in two 24-week trials conducted in obese patients with type 2 diabetes, bromocriptine in combination with sulfonylurea therapy resulted in a 0.55% reduction in HbA_{1c} in comparison to placebo plus sulfonylureas (The Pink Sheet, May 18, 1998). In addition, a study conducted in 159 type 2 patients found that monotherapy with bromocriptine resulted in a reduction in HbA_{1c} of 0.44% in comparison to placebo. The sponsor has advocated the use of a responder approach to screen out poor responders and thereby increase the average response among those patients who remain on therapy.

CONCLUSIONS

The achievement and maintenance of euglycemia remains an elusive goal for many diabetic patients. In particular, monotherapy appears to be inadequate for the long-term treatment of many patients with type 2 diasease.   However, several novel approaches to the improvement of glycemic control have demonstrated promise, and the expanded options available to both type 1 and type 2 diabetic patients represent a significant advance in the treatment of these diseases. With conclusive evidence linking improved glycemic control to a reduction in microvascular complications, the importance of developing effective therapies to achieve this goal cannot be overstated.

References

Abbott WG, Boyce VL, Grundy SM, Howard BV. Effects of replacing saturated fat with complex carbohydrate in diets of subjects with NIDDM. *Diabetes Care* 1989; **12**(2): 102–107.

Agurs-Collins TD, Kumanyika SK, Ten Have TR, Adams-Campbell LL. A randomized controlled trial of weight reduction and exercise for diabetes management in older African-American subjects. *Diabetes Care* 1997; **20**(10): 1503–1511.

al-Achi A, Greenwood R. Buccal administration of human insulin in streptozotocin-diabetic rats. *Res Commun Chem Pathol Pharmacol* 1993; **82**(3): 297–306.

American Diabetes Association. Nutritional recommendations and principles for individuals with diabetes mellitus [position statement]. *Diabetes Care* 1997; **20**(Suppl 1): 15–18.

American Diabetes Association. The pharmacological treatment of hyperglycemia in NIDDM [consensus statement]. *Diabetes Care* 1996; **19**(Suppl 1): 54–61.

Anderson JH Jr, Brunelle RL, Keohane P, Koivisto VA, Trautmann ME, Vignati L, DiMarchi R. Mealtime treatment with insulin analog improves postprandial hyperglycemia and hypoglycemia in patients with non-insulin-dependent diabetes mellitus. Multicenter Insulin Lispro Study Group. *Arch Intern Med* 1997b; **157**(11): 1249–1255.

Anderson JH Jr., Brunelle RL, Koivisto VA, Pfutzner A, Trautmann ME, Vignati L, DiMarchi R. Reduction of postprandial hyperglycemia and frequency of hypoglycemia in IDDM patients on insulin-analog treatment. Multicenter Insulin Lispro Study Group. *Diabetes* 1997a; **46**(2): 265–270.

Antonucci T, Whitcomb R, McLain R, Lockwood D, Norris RM. Impaired glucose tolerance is normalized by treatment with the thiazolidinedione troglitazone. *Diabetes Care* 1997; **20**(2): 188–193.

Atkinson PR, Mahon JL, Bupre J, Stiller CR, Jenner MR, Paul TL, Momah CI. Interaction of bromocriptine and cyclosporine in insulin dependent diabetes mellitus: results from the Canadian open study. *J Autoimmun* 1990; **3**(6): 793–799.

Aungst BJ, Rogers NJ, Shefter E. Comparison of nasal, rectal, buccal, sublingual, and intramuscular insulin efficacy and the effects of bile salt absorption promoter. *J Pharmacol Exp Ther* 1988; **244**(1): 23–27.

Bailey CJ. Biguanides and NIDDM. *Diabetes Care* 1992; **15**(6): 755–772.

Bakkali-Nadi A, Malaisse-Lagae F, Malaisse WJ. Insulinotropic action of meglitinide analogs: concentration-response relationship and nutrient dependency. *Diabetes Res* 1994; **27**(2): 81–87.

Balfour JA, Faulds D. Repaglinide. *Drugs Aging* 1998; **13**(2): 173–180.

Barnett AH, Chapman C, Gailer K, Hayter CJ. Effect of bromocriptine on maturity onset diabetes. *Postgrad Med J* 1980; **56**(651): 11–14.

Barnett AH, Owens DR. Insulin analogues. *Lancet* 1997; **349**: 47–51.

Bartlett JD, Turner-Henson A, Atchison JA, Woolley TW, Pillion DJ. Insulin administration to the eyes of normoglycemic human volunteers. *J Ocul Pharmacol* 1994; **10**(4): 683–690.

Berkowitz K, Peters R, Kjos SL, Goico J, Marroquin A, Dunn ME, Xiang A, Azen S, Buchanan TA. Effect of troglitazone on insulin sensitivity and pancreatic beta-cell function in women at high risk for NIDDM. *Diabetes* 1996; **45**(11): 1572–1579.

Bernkop-Schnurch A. The use of inhibitory agents to overcome the enzymatic barrier to perorally administered therapeutic peptides and proteins. *J Controlled Release* 1998; **52**(1–2): 1–16.

Berti L, Kellerer M, Bossenmaier B, Seffer E, Seipke G, Haring HU. The long acting human insulin analog HOE 901: characteristics of insulin signaling in comparison to Asp (B10) and regular insulin. *Horm Metab Res* 1998; **30**(3): 123–129.

Binder C, Lauritzen T, Faber O, Pramming S. Insulin pharmacokinetics. *Diabetes Care* 1984; **7**: 188–199.

Bode BW, Steed RD, Davidson PC. Reduction in severe hypoglycemia with long-term continuous subcutaneous insulin infusion in type 1 diabetes. *Diabetes Care* 1996; **19**(4): 324–327.

Bornfeldt KE, Gidlöf RA, Wasteson A, Lake M, Skottner A, Arnqvist HJ. Binding and biological effects of insulin, insulin analogues, and insulin-like growth factors in rat aortic smooth muscle cells: comparison of maximal growth promoting activities. *Diabetologia* 1991; **34**: 307–313.

Brady PA, Terzic A. The sulfonylurea controversy: more questions from the heart. *J Am Coll Cardiol* 1998; **31**(5): 950–956.

Braun B, Zimmermann MB, Kretchmer N. Effects of exercise intensity on insulin sensitivity in women with non-insulin-dependent diabetes mellitus. *J Appl Physiol* 1995; **78**(1): 300–306.

Bruce DG, Chisholm DJ, Storlien LH, Borkman M, Kraegen EW. Meal-time intranasal insulin delivery in type 2 diabetes. *Diabet Med* 1991; **8**(4): 366–370.

Bruttomesso D, Biolo G, Inchiostro S, Fongher C, Briani G, Duner E, Marescotti MC, Iori E, Tiengo A, Tessari P. No effects of high-fiber diets on metabolic control and insulin-sensitivity in type 1 diabetic subjects. *Diabetes Res Clin Pract* 1991; **13**(1–2): 15–21.

Califano J. Order of the secretary, U.S. Department of Health, Education, and Welfare, Suspending Approval. *Re: New Drug Applications for Phenformin: NDA 11-624, NDA 12-752, NDA 17-127*; 17 July, 1977.

Campbell LV, Marmot PE, Dyer JA, Borkman M, Storlien LH. The high-monounsaturated fat diet as a practical alternative for NIDDM. *Diabetes Care* 1994; **17**(3): 177–182.

Campbell RK, Campbell LK, White JR. Insulin lispro: its role in the treatment of diabetes mellitus. *Ann Pharmacother* 1996; **30**: 1263–1271.

Cavaghan MK, Ehrmann DA, Byrne MM, Polonsky KS. Treatment with the oral antidiabetic agent troglitazone improves beta cell responses to glucose in subjects with impaired glucose tolerance. *J Clin Invest* 1997; **100**(3): 530–537.

Cheng CL, Gehrke SH, Ritschel WA. Development of an azopolymer based colonic release capsule for delivering proteins/macromolecules. *Methods Find Exp Clin Pharmacol* 1994; **16**(4): 271–278.

Chiasson JL, Josse RG, Hynt JA, Palmason C, Rodger NW, Ross SA, Ryan EA, Tan MH, Wolever TM. The efficacy of acarbose in the treatment of patients with non-insulin-dependent diabetes mellitus. A multicenter controlled clinical trial. *Ann Intern Med* 1994; **121**(12): 928–935.

Cincotta AH, Meier AH, Southern LL. Bromocriptine alters hormone rhythms and lipid metabolism in swine. *Ann Nutr Metab* 1989; **33**(6): 305–314.

Cincotta AH, MacEachern TA, Meier AH. Bromocriptine redirects metabolism and prevents seasonal onset of obese hyperinsulinemic state in Syrian hamsters. *Am J Physiol* 1993; **264**(2 Pt 1): E285–E293.

Cincotta AH, Schiller BC, Meier AH. Bromocriptine inhibits the seasonally occurring obesity, hyperinsulinemia, insulin resistance, and impaired glucose tolerance in the Syrian hamster, Mesocricetus auratus. *Metabolism* 1991; **40**(6): 639–644.

Cleveland JC Jr., Meldrum DR, Cain BS, Banerjee A, Harken AH. Oral sulfonylurea hypoglycemic agents prevent ischemic preconditioning in human myocardium. Two paradoxes revisited. *Circulation* 1997; **96**(1): 29–32.

Clinical Investigator News. *Endocrinology.* July, 1998; **6**(7): 9.

Coates PA, Ismail IS, Luzio SD, Griffiths I, Ollerton RL, Volund A, Owens DR. Intranasal insulin: the effects of three dose regimens on postprandial glycaemic profiles in type II diabetic subjects. *Diabet Med* 1995b; **12**(3): 235–239.

Coates PA, Mukherjee S, Luzio S, et al. Pharmacokinetics of a "long-acting" human insulin analog (HOE901) in healthy subjects. *Diabetes* 1995a; **44**(Suppl 1): 130A.

Coniff RF, Shapiro JA, Robbins D, Kleinfeld R, Seaton TB, Beisswenger P, McGill JB. Reduction of glycosylated hemoglobin and postprandial hyperglycemia by acarbose in patients with NIDDM. A placebo-controlled dose-comparison study. *Diabetes Care* 1995b; **18**(6): 817–824.

Coniff RF, Shapiro JA, Seaton TB, Bray GA. Multicenter, placebo-controlled trial comparing acarbose (BAY g 5421) with placebo, tolbutamide, and tolbutamide-plus-acarbose in non-insulin-dependent diabetes mellitus. *Am J Med* 1995a; **98**(5): 443–451.

Coniff RF, Shapiro JA, Seaton TB, Hoogwerf BJ, Hunt JA. A double-blind placebo-controlled trial evaluating the safety and efficacy of acarbose for the treatment of patients with insulin-requiring type II diabetes. *Diabetes Care* 1995c; **18**(7): 928–932.

Damage C, Vranckx H, Balshmidt P, Couvreur P. Poly (alkyl cyanoacrylate) nanospheres for oral administration of insulin. *J Pharm Sci* 1997; **86**(12): 1403–1409.

Daniels AR, Bruce R, McGregor L. Lispro insulin as premeal therapy in type 1 diabetes: comparison with Humulin R. *N Z Med J* 1997; **110**(1056): 435–438.

Davey P, Grainger D, MacMillan J, Rajan N, Aristides M, Gliksman M. Clinical outcomes with insulin lispro compared with human regular insulin: a meta-analysis. *Clin Ther* 1997; **19**(4): 656–674.

Davidson MB, Peters AL. An overview of metformin in the treatment of type 2 diabetes mellitus. *Am J Med* 1997; **102**(1): 99–110.

DCCT Research Group. The effect of intensive treatment of diabetes on the development and progression of long-term complications in insulin-dependent diabetes mellitus. *N Engl J Med* 1993; **329**(14): 977–986.

DCCT Research Group. The absence of a glycemic threshold for the development of long-term complications: the perspective of the Diabetes Control and Complications Trial. *Diabetes* 1996; **45**: 1289–1298.

Dolocek R, Kubis M, Sajnar J, Zavada M. Bromocriptine and glucose tolerance in acromegalics. *Pharmatherapeutica* 1982; **3**(2): 100–106.

Draeger E. Clinical profile of glimepiride. *Diabetes Res Clin Pract* 1995; **28**(Suppl): S139–S146.

Drejer K. The bioactivity of insulin analogues from in vitro receptor binding to in vivo glucose uptake. *Diabetes Metab Rev* 1992; **8**: 259–285.

Drejer K, Vaag A, Bech K, Hansen P, Sorensen AR, Mygind N. Intranasal administration of insulin with phospholipid as absorption enhancer: pharmacokinetics in normal subjects. *Diabet Med* 1992; **9**(4): 335–340.

Dunn FL, Nathan DM, Scavini M, Selam JL, Wingrove TG. Long-term therapy of IDDM with an implantable insulin pump. The Implantable Insulin Pump Trial Study Group. *Diabetes Care* 1997; **20**(1): 59–63.

Edwards DA, Hanes J, Caponetti G, Hrkach J, Ben-Jebria A, Eskew ML, Mintzes J, Deaver D, Lotan N, Langer R. Large porous particles for pulmonary drug delivery. *Science* 1997; **276**: 1868–1871.

Flint A, Raben A, Astrup A, Holst JJ. Glucagon-like peptide 1 promotes satiety and suppresses energy intake in humans. *J Clin Invest* 1998; **101**(3): 515–520.

Frauman AG, Cooper ME, Parsons BJ, Jerums G, Louis WJ. Long-term use of intranasal insulin in insulin-dependent diabetic patients. *Diabetes Care* 1987; **10**(5): 573–578.

Fuhlendorff J, Rorsman P, Kofod H, Brand CL, Rolin B, MacKay P, Shymko R, Carr RD. Simulation of insulin release by repaglinide and glibenclamide involves both common and distinct processes. *Diabetes* 1998; **47**(3): 345–351.

Garg A. High-monounsaturated-fat diets for patients with diabetes mellitus: a meta-analysis. *Am J Clin Nutr* 1998; **67**(3 Suppl): 577–582.

Garg A, Bantle JP, Henry RR, Coulston AM, Griver KA, Raatz SK, Brinkley L, Chen YD, Grundy SM, Huet BA, et al. Effects of varying carbohydrate content of diet in patients with non-insulin-dependent diabetes mellitus. *JAMA* 1994; **271**(18): 1421–1428.

Garg A, Grundy SM, Unger RH. Comparison of effects of high and low carbohydrate diets on plasma lipoproteins and insulin sensitivity in patients with mild NIDDM. *Diabetes* 1992; **41**(10): 1278–1285.

Gerich JE. Oral hypoglycemic agents. *N Engl J Med* 1989; **321**(18): 1231–1245.

Ghazzi MN, Perez JE, Antonucci TK, Driscoll JH, Huang SM, Faja BW, Troglitazone Study Group, Whitcomb RW. Cardiac and glycemic benefits of troglitazone treatment in NIDDM. *Diabetes* 1997; **46**: 433–439.

Gittelsohn J, Wolever TM, Harris SB, Harris-Giraldo R, Hanley AJ, Zinman B. Specific patterns of food consumption and preparation are associated with diabetes and obesity in a Native Canadian community. *J Nutr* 1998; **128**(3): 541–547.

Goodyear LJ, Kahn BB. Exercise, glucose transport, and insulin sensitivity. *Ann Rev Med* 1998; **49**: 235–261.

Graff MR, McClanahan MA. Assessment by patients with diabetes mellitus of two insulin pen delivery systems versus a vial and syringe. *Clin Ther* 1998; **20**(3): 486–496.

Greenfield MS, Doberne L, Rosenthal M, Schulz B, Widstrom A, Reaven GM. Effect of sulfonylurea treatment on in vivo insulin secretion and action in patients with non-insulin-dependent diabetes mellitus. *Diabetes* 1982; **31**(4 Part 1): 307–312.

Gwinup G, Elias AN, Domurat ES. Insulin and C-peptide levels following oral administration of insulin in intestinal-enzyme protected capsules. *Gen Pharmacol* 1991; **22**(2): 243–246.

Hawkins TA, Gala RR, Dunbar JC. Prolactin modulates the incidence of diabetes in male and female NOD mice. *Autoimmunity* 1994; **18**(3): 155–162.

Heinemann L, Traut T, Heise T. Time-action profile of inhaled insulin. *Diabet Med* 1997; **14**(1): 63–72.

Henry RR. Thiazolidinediones. *Endocrinol Metab Clin North Am* 1997; **26**(3): 553–573.

Hermans MP, van Ypersele de Strihou M, Ketelslegers JM, Squifflet JP, Buysschaert M. Fasting and postprandial plasma glucose and peripheral insulin levels in insulin-dependent diabetes mellitus and non-insulin-dependent diabetes mellitus subjects during continuous intraperitoneal versus subcutaneous insulin delivery. *Transplant Proc* 1995; **27**(6): 3329–3330.

Hilsted J, Madsbad S, Hvidberg A, Rasmussen MH, Krarup T, Ipsen H, Hansen B, Pedersen M, Djurup R, Oxenboll B. Intranasal insulin therapy: the clinical realities. *Diabetologia* 1995; **38**(6): 680–684.

Hoffman A, Ziv E. Pharmacokinetic considerations of new insulin formulations and routes of administration. *Clin Pharmacokinet* 1997; **33**(4): 285–301.

Hoffmann J, Spengler M. Efficacy of 24-week monotherapy with acarbose, metformin, or placebo in dietary-treated NIDDM patients: the Essen-II Study. *Am J Med* 1997; **103**(6): 483–490.

Hollander P, Pi-Sunyer X, Coniff RF. Acarbose in the treatment of type 1 diabetes. *Diabetes Care* 1997; **20**(3): 248–253.

Holleman F, Hoekstra JBL. Insulin lispro. *N Engl J Med* 1997; **337**(3): 176–183.

Holleman F, Schmitt H, Rottiers R, Rees A, Symanowski S, Anderson JH. Reduced frequency of severe hypoglycemia and coma in well-controlled IDDM patients treated with insulin lispro. *Diabetes Care* 1997; **20**(12): 1827–1832.

Hollenbeck CB, Johnston P, Varasteh BB, Chen YD, Reaven GM. Effects of metformin on glucose, insulin and lipid metabolism in patients with mild hypertriglyceridaemia and non-insulin dependent diabetes by glucose tolerance test criteria. *Diabete Metab* 1991; **17**(5): 483–489.

Howard BV, Abbott WG, Swinburn BA. Evaluation of metabolic effects of substitution of complex carbohydrates for saturated fat in individuals with obesity and NIDDM. *Diabetes Care* 1991; **14**(9): 786–795.

Inoue I, Takahashi K, Noji S, Awata T, Negishi K, Katayama S. Acarbose controls postprandial hyperproinsulinemia in non-insulin-dependent diabetes mellitus. *Diabetes Res Clin Pract* 1997; **36**(3): 143–151.

Ishii T, Yamakita T, Sato T, Tanaka S, Fujii S. Resistance training improves insulin sensitivity in NIDDM subjects without altering maximal oxygen uptake. *Diabetes Care* 1998; **21**(8): 1353–1355.

Iwamoto Y, Kosaka K, Kuzuya T, Akanuma Y, Shigeta Y, Kaneko T. Effects of troglitazone: a new hypoglycemic agent in patients with NIDDM poorly controlled by diet therapy. *Diabetes Care* 1996; **19**: 151–156.

Iwamoto Y, Kuzuya T, Matsuda A, Awata T, Kumakara S, Inooka G, Shiraishi I. Effect of new oral antidiabetic agent CS-045 on glucose tolerance and insulin secretion in patients with NIDDM. *Diabetes Care* 1991; **14**(11): 1083–1086.

Jacobs MA, Schreuder RH, Jap-A-Joe K, Nauta JJ, Andersen PM, Heine RJ. The pharmacodynamics and activity of intranasally administered insulin in healthy male volunteers. *Diabetes* 1993; **42**(11): 1649–1655.

Janssen MM, Casteleijn S, Deville W, Popp-Snijders C, Roach P, Heine RJ. Nighttime insulin kinetics and glycemic control in type 1 diabetes patients following administration of an intermediate-acting lispro preparation. *Diabetes Care* 1997; **20**(12): 1870–1873.

Jendle JH, Karlberg BE. Intrapulmonary administration of insulin to healthy volunteers. *J Intern Med* 1996a; **240**(2): 93–98.

Jendle JH, Karlberg BE. Effects of intrapulmonary insulin in patients with non-insulin-dependent diabetes. *Scand J Clin Lab Invest* 1996b; **56**(6): 555–561.

Jennings AM, Lewis KS, Murdoch S, Talbot JF, Bradley C, Ward JD. Randomized trial comparing continuous subcutaneous insulin infusion and conventional insulin therapy in type II diabetic patients poorly controlled with sulfonylureas. *Diabetes Care* 1991; **14**(8): 738–744.

Johnson MD, Campbell LK, Campbell RK. Troglitazone: review and assessment of its role in the treatment of patients with impaired glucose tolerance and diabetes mellitus. *Ann*

Pharmacother 1998; **32**(3): 337–348.

Johnston PS, Coniff RF, Hoogwerf BJ, Santiago JV, Pi-Sunyer FX, Krol A. Effects of the carbohydrase inhibitor miglitol in sulfonylurea-treated NIDDM patients. *Diabetes Care* 1994; **17**(1): 20–29.

Jorgensen S, Vaag A, Langkjaer L, Hougaard P, Markussen J. NovoSol Basal: pharmacokinetics of a novel soluble long-acting insulin analogue. *BMJ* 1989; **299**(6696): 415–419.

Kanc K, Janssen MM, Keulen ET, Jacobs MA, Popp-Snijders C, Snoek FJ, Heine RJ. Substitution of nighttime continuous subcutaneous insulin infusion therapy for bedtime NPH insulin in a multiple injection regimen improves counter-regulatory hormonal responses and warning symptoms of hypoglycemia in IDDM. *Diabetologia* 1998; **41**(3): 322–329.

Kang S, Brange J, Burch A, Volund A, Owens DR. Subcutaneous insulin absorption explained by insulin's physicochemical properties. Evidence from absorption studies of soluble human insulin and insulin analogues in humans. *Diabetes Care* 1991a; **14**(11): 942–948.

Kang S, Creagh FM, Peters JR, Brange J, Vølund A, Owens DR. Comparison of subcutaneous soluble human insulin and insulin analogues (Asp^{B9}; Glu^{B27}; Asp^{B10}; Asp^{B28}) on meal-related plasma glucose excursions in type I diabetic subjects. *Diabetes Care* 1991b; **14**: 571–577.

Kelley DE, Henry RR, Edelman SV, Veterans Affairs Implantable Insulin Pump Study Group. Acute effects of intraperitoneal versus subcutaneous insulin delivery on glucose homeostasis in patients with NIDDM. *Diabetes Care* 1996; **19**(11): 1237–1242.

Kikuchi M. Modulation of insulin secretion in non-insulin-dependent diabetes mellitus by two novel oral hypoglycemic agents, NN623 and A4166. *Diabet Med* 1996; **13**(Suppl 6): S151–S155.

Kostanos JG, Vignati L, Huster W, Andrejasich C, Boggs MB, Jacobson AM, Marrero D, Mathias SD, Patrick D, Zalani S, et al. Health-related quality-of-life results from multinational clinical trials of insulin lispro. Assessing benefits of a new diabetes therapy. *Diabetes Care* 1997; **20**(6): 948–958.

Kumar S, Boulton AJ, Beck-Nielsen H, Berthezene F, Muggeo M, Persson B, Spinas GA, Donoghue S, Lettis S, Stewart-Long P. Troglitazone, an insulin action enhancer, improves metabolic control in NIDDM patients. Troglitazone Study Group. *Diabetologia* 1996; **39**(6): 701–709.

Lambe KG, Tugwood JD. A human peroxisome-proliferator-activated receptor-gamma is activated by inducers of adipogenesis, including thiazolidinedione drugs. *Eur J Biochem* 1996; **239**(1): 1–7.

Langtry HD, Balfour JA. Glimepiride. A review of its use in the management of type 2 diabetes mellitus. *Drugs* 1998; **55**(4): 563–584.

Laube BL, Georopoulos A, Adams GK 3rd. Preliminary study of the efficacy of insulin aerosol delivered by oral inhalation in diabetic patients. *JAMA* 1993; **269**(16): 2106–2109.

Lean MEJ, Ng LL, Tennison BR. Interval between insulin injection and eating in relation to blood glucose control in adult diabetics. *BMJ* 1985; **290**: 105–108.

Lehmann R, Kaplan V, Bingisser R, Bloch KE, Spinas GA. Impact of physical activity on cardiovascular risk factors in IDDM. *Diabetes Care* 1997; **20**(10): 1603–1611.

Levy J, Atkinson AB, Bell PM, McCance DR, Hadden DR. Beta-cell deterioration determines the onset and rate of progression of secondary dietary failure in type 2 diabetes mellitus: the 10-year follow-up of the Belfast Diet Study. *Diabet Med* 1998; **15**(4): 290–296.

Liang Y, Jetton TL, Lubkin M, Meier AH, Cincotta AH. Bromocriptine/ SKF38393 ameliorates islet dysfunction in the diabetic (db/db) mouse. *Cell Mol Life Sci* 1998; **54**(7): 703–711.

Macdonald IA. Amylin and the gastrointestinal tract. *Diabet Med* 1997; **14**(Suppl 2): S24–S28.

Maggs DG, Buchanan TA, Burant CF, Cline G, Gumbiner B, Hsueh WA, Inzucchi S, Kelley D, Nolan J, Olefsky JM, Polonsky KS, Silver D, Valiquett TR, Shulman GI. Metabolic effects of troglitazone monotherapy in type 2 diabetes mellitus. A randomized, double-blind, placebo-controlled trial. *Ann Intern Med* 1998; **128**(3): 176–185.

Markussen J, Havelund S, Kurtzhals P, Andersen AS, Halstrom J, Hasselager E, Larsen UD, Ribel U, Schaffer L, Vad K, et al. Soluble, fatty acid acylated insulins bind to albumin and show protracted action in pigs. *Diabetologia* 1996; **39**(3): 281–288.

Marshall JA, Bessesen DH, Hamman RF. High saturated fat and low starch and fibre are associated with hyperinsulinaemia in a non-diabetic population: the San Luis Valley Diabetes Study. *Diabetologia* 1997; **40**(4): 430–438.

Marshall JA, Hoag S, Shetterly S, Hamman RF. Dietary fat predicts conversion from impaired glucose tolerance to NIDDM. The San Luis Valley Diabetes Study. *Diabetes Care* 1994; **17**(1): 50–56.

Marshall SM, Home PD, Taylor R, Alberti KG. Continuous subcutaneous insulin infusion versus injection therapy: a randomized cross-over trial under usual diabetic clinic conditions. *Diabet Med* 1987; **4**(6): 521–525.

Mayer-Davis EJ, D'Agostino R Jr, Karter AJ, Haffner SM, Rewers MJ, Saad M, Bergman RN. Intensity and amount of physical activity in relation to insulin sensitivity: the Insulin Resistance Atherosclerosis Study. *JAMA* 1998; **279**(9): 669–674.

Meier AH, Cincotta AH, Lovell WC. Timed bromocriptine administration reduces body fat stores in obese subjects and hyperglycemia in type II diabetics. *Experientia* 1992; **48**(3): 248–253.

Meinert CL, Knatterud GL, Prout TE, Klimt CR. A study of the effects of hypoglycemic agents on vascular complications in patients with adult-onset diabetes. II. Mortality results. *Diabetes* 1970; **19**(Suppl): 789–830.

Melander A, Bitzen PO, Faber O, Groop L. Sulphonylurea antidiabetic drugs. An update of their clinical pharmacology and rational therapeutic use. *Drugs* 1989; **37**(1): 58–72.

Melchior WR, Jaber LA. Metformin: an anti-hyperglycemic agent for treatment of type II diabetes. *Ann Pharmacother* 1996; **30**(2): 158–164.

Melki V, Renard E, Lassmann-Vague V, Boivin S, Guerci B, Hanaire-Broutin H, Bringer J, Belicar P, Jeandidier N, Meyer L, et al. Improvement of HbA$_{1c}$ and blood glucose stability in IDDM patients treated with lispro insulin analog in external pumps. *Diabetes Care* 1998; **21**(6): 977–982.

Minamikawa J, Tanaka S, Yamauchi M, Inoue D, Koshiyama H. Potent inhibitory effect of troglitazone on carotid arterial wall thickness in type 2 diabetes. *J Endocrinol Metab* 1998; **83**(5): 1818–1820.

Mooradian AD, Morley JE, Billington CJ, Slag MF, Elson MK, Shafer RB. Hyperprolactinaemia in male diabetics. *Postgrad Med J* 1985; **61**(711): 11–14.

Mosher PE, Nash MS, Perry AC, LaPerriere AR, Goldberg RB. Aerobic circuit exercise training: effect on adolescents with well-controlled insulin-dependent diabetes mellitus. *Arch Phys Med Rehabil* 1998; **79**(6): 652–657.

Myers SR, Yakubu-Madus FE, Johnson WT, Baker JE, Cusick TS, Williams VK, Tinsley FC, Kriauciunas A, Manetta J, Chen VJ. Acylation of human insulin with palmitic acid extends the time action of human insulin in diabetic dogs. *Diabetes* 1997; **46**(4): 637–642.

Naslund E, Gutniak M, Skogar S, Rossner S, Hellstrom PM. Glucagon-like peptide 1 increases the period of postprandial satiety and slows gastric emptying in obese men. *Am J Clin Nutr* 1998; **68**(3): 525–530.

Nathan DM, Schreiber E, Fogel H, Mosjov S, Habener JF. Insulinotropic action of glucagon peptide-1-(7–37) in diabetic and nondiabetic subjects. *Diabetes Care* 1992; **15**(2): 270–276.

Nauck MA, Kleine N, Orskov C, Holst JJ, Willms B, Creutzfeldt W. Normalization of fasting hyperglycemia by exogenous glucagon-like peptide 1 (7–36 amide) in type 2 (non-insulin-dependent) diabetic patients. *Diabetologia* 1993; **36**(8): 741–744.

Nauck MA, Sauerwald A, Ritzel R, Holst JJ, Schmiegel W. Influence of glucagon-like peptide 1 on fasting glycaemia in type 2 diabetic patients treated with insulin after sulfonylurea secondary failure. *Diabetes Care* 1998a; **21**(11): 1925–1931.

Nauck MA, Weber I, Bach I, Richter S, Orskov C, Holst JJ, Schmiegel W. Normalization of fasting glycaemia by intravenous GLP-1 ([7–36 amide] or [7–37]) in type 2 diabetic patients. *Diabet Med* 1998b; **15**(11): 937–945.

Nielsen FS, Jorgensen LN, Ipsen M, Voldsgaard AI, Parving HH. Long-term comparison of human insulin analogue B10Asp and soluble human insulin in IDDM patients on a basal/bolus insulin regimen. *Diabetologia* 1995; **38**(5): 592–598.

Nishihata T, Kamada A, Sakai K, Yagi T, Kawamori R, Shichiri M. Effectiveness of insulin suppositories in diabetic patients. *J Pharm Pharmacol* 1989; **4**: 799–801.

Nolan JJ, Ludvik B, Beerdsen P, Joyce M, Olefsky J. Improvement in glucose tolerance and insulin resistance in obese subjects treated with troglitazone. *N Engl J Med* 1994; **331**(18): 1188–1193.

Ogihara T, Rakugi H, Ikegami H, Mikami H, Masuo K. Enhancement of insulin sensitivity by troglitazone lowers blood pressure in diabetic hypertensives. *Am J Hypertens* 1995; **8**(3): 316–320.

Oh CK, Ritschel WA. Absorption characteristics of insulin through the buccal mucosa. *Methods Find Exp Clin Pharmacol* 1990; **12**(4): 275–279.

Ohkubo Y, Kishikawa H, Araki E, Miyata T, Isami S, Motoyoshi S, Kojima Y. Furuyoshi N, Shichiri M. Intensive insulin treatment prevents the progression of diabetic microvascular complications in Japanese patients with non-insulin-dependent diabetes mellitus: a randomized prospective 6-year study. *Diabetes Res Clin Pract* 1995; **28**(2): 103–117.

Olsen CL, Liu G, Iravani M, Nguyen S, Khourdadjian K, Turner DS, Waxman K, Selam JL, Charles MA. Long-term safety and efficacy of programmable implantable insulin delivery systems. *Int J Artif Organs* 1993; **16**(12): 847–854.

Olsson PO, Arnqvist HJ, Von Schenk HV. Free insulin profiles during intensive treatment with biosynthetic human insulin. *Diabete Metab* 1988; **14**(3): 253–258.

Paisey RB, Harvey P, Rice S, Belka I, Bower L, Dunn M, Taylor P, Paisey RM, Frost J, Ash I. An intensive weight loss programme in established type 2 diabetes and controls: effects on weight and atherosclerosis risk factors at one year. *Diabet Med* 1998; **15**(1): 73–79.

Palumbo PJ. Metformin: effects on cardiovascular risk factors in patients with non-insulin-dependent diabetes mellitus. *J Diabetes Complications* 1998; **12**(2): 110–119.

Pfutzner A, Kustner E, Forst T, Schulze-Schleppinghoff B, Trautmann ME, Haslbeck M, Schatz H, Beyer J. Intensive insulin therapy with insulin lispro in patients with type 1 diabetes reduces the frequency of hypoglycemic episodes. *Exp Clin Endocrinol Diabetes* 1996; **104**(1): 25–30.

Pick ME, Hawrysh ZJ, Gee MI, Toth E, Garg ML, Hardin RT. Oat bran concentrate bread products improve long-term control of diabetes: a pilot study. *J Am Diet Assoc* 1996; **96**(12): 1254–1261.

The Pink Sheet. Ergo *Ergoset* systemic effects need further examination - FDA cmte. May 18, 1998, p. 8.

Prendergast BD. Glyburide and glipizide, second generation oral sulfonylurea hypoglycemic agents. *Clin Pharm* 1984; **3**(5): 473–485.

Prigeon RL, Kahn SE, Porte D Jr. Effect of troglitazone on β cell function, insulin sensitivity, and glycemic control in subjects with type 2 diabetes mellitus. *J Clin Endocrinol Metab* 1998; **83**(3): 819–823.

Qualmann C, Nauck MA, Holst JJ, Orskov C, Creutzfeldt W. Insulinotropic actions of intravenous glucagon-like peptide-1 (GLP-1) [7–36 amide] in the fasting state in healthy subjects. *Acta Diabetol* 1995; **32**(1): 13–16.

Renard E, Baldet P, Picot MC, Jacques-Apostol D, Lauton D, Costalat G, Bringer J, Jaffiol C. Catheter complications associated with implantable systems for peritoneal insulin delivery. An analysis of frequency, predisposing factors, and obstructing materials. *Diabetes Care* 1995; **18**(3): 300–306.

Riccardi G, Rivallese AA. Effects of dietary fiber and carbohydrate on glucose and lipoprotein metabolism in diabetic patients. *Diabetes Care* 1991; **14**(12): 1115–1125.

Rios MS. Acarbose and insulin therapy in type I diabetes mellitus. *Eur J Clin Invest* 1994; **24**(Suppl 3): 36–39.

Rojdmark S, Rossner S. Decreased dopaminergic control of prolactin secretion in male obesity: normalization by fasting. *Metabolism* 1991; **40**(2): 191–195.

Saffran M, Field JB, Pena J, Jones RH, Okuda Y. Oral insulin in diabetic dogs. *J Endocrinol* 1991; **131**(2): 267–278.

Santeusanio F, Compagnucci P. A risk-benefit appraisal of acarbose in the management of non-insulin-dependent diabetes mellitus. *Drug Saf* 1994; **11**(6): 432–444.

Saudek CD. Novel forms of insulin delivery. *Endocrinol Metab Clin North Am* 1997; **26**(3): 599–610.

Saudek CD, Duckworth WC, Giobbie-Hurder A, Henderson WG, Henry RR, Kelley DE, Edelman SV, Zieve FJ, Adler RA, Anderson JW, et al. Implantable insulin pump vs multiple-dose insulin for non-insulin-dependent diabetes mellitus: a randomized clinical trial. Department of Veterans Affairs Implantable Insulin Pump Study Group. *JAMA* 1996; **276**(16): 1322–1327.

Scheen AJ. Drug treatment of non-insulin-dependent diabetes mellitus in the 1990s. Achievements and future developments. *Drugs* 1997; **54**(3): 355–368.

Scheen AJ, Lefebvre PJ. Oral antidiabetic agents. A guide to selection. *Drugs* 1998; **55**(2): 225–236.

Scherbaum WA. The role of amylin in the physiology of glycemic control. *Exp Clin Endocrinol Diabetes* 1998; **102**(2): 97–102.

Schernthaner G. Immunogenicity and allergenic potential of animal and human insulins. *Diabetes Care* 1993; **16**(Suppl 3): 155–165.

Schiffrin A, Belmonte MM. Comparison between continuous subcutaneous insulin infusion and multiple injections of insulin. A one-year prospective study. *Diabetes* 1982; **31**(3): 255–264.

Schirra J, Leicht P, Hildebrand P, Beglinger C, Arnold R, Goke B, Katschinski M. Mechanisms of the antidiabetic action of subcutaneous glucagon-like peptide-1 (7–36) amide in non-insulin dependent diabetes mellitus. *J Endocrinol* 1998; **156**(1): 177–186.

Schneider SH, Amorosa LF, Khachadurian AK, Ruderman NB. Studies on the mechanism of improved glucose control during regular exercise in type 2 (non-insulin-dependent) diabetes. *Diabetologia* 1984; **26**(5): 355–360.

Schwartz S, Raskin P, Fonseca V, Graveline JF. Effect of troglitazone in insulin-treated patients with type II diabetes mellitus. Troglitazone and Exogenous Insulin Study Group. *N Engl J Med* 1998; **338**(13): 861–866.

Scobie IN, Kesson CM, Ratcliffe JG, Maccuish AC. The effects of prolonged bromocriptine administration on PRL secretion, GH, and glycaemic control in stable insulin-dependent diabetes mellitus. *Clin Endocrinol (Oxf)* 1983; **18**(2): 179–185.

Scrip No. 2279. Inhale seeks additional partners. October 28, 1997; p. 13.

Scrip No. 2345. 1st Phase II results on inhaled insulin. June 19, 1998, p. 21.

Serrano-Rios M, Saban J, Navascues I, Canizo JF, Hillebrand I. Effect of two new alpha-glucosidase inhibitors in insulin-dependent diabetic patients. *Diabetes Res Clin Pract* 1988; **4**(2): 111–116.

Service RF. Drug delivery takes a deep breath. *Science* 1997; **277**(5330): 1199–1200.

Shen HQ, Roth MD, Peterson RG. The effect of glucose and glucagon-like peptide-1 stimulation on insulin release in the perfused pancreas in a non-insulin-dependent diabetes mellitus animal model. *Metabolism* 1998; **47**(9): 1042–1047.

Shorr RI, Ray WA, Daugherty JR, Griffin MR. Individual sulfonylureas and serious hypoglycemia in older people. *J Am Geriatr Soc* 1996; **44**(7): 751–755.

Sironi AM, Vichi S, Gastaldelli A, Pecori N, Anichini R, Foot E, Seghieri G, Ferrannini E. Effects of troglitazone on insulin action and cardiovascular risk factors in patients with non-insulin-dependent diabetes mellitus. *Clin Pharmacol Ther* 1997; **62**(2): 194–202.

Skillman CA, Raskin P. A double-masked placebo-controlled trial assessing effects of various doses of BTS 67,582, a novel insulinotropic agent, on fasting hyperglycemia in NIDDM patients. *Diabetes Care* 1997; **20**(4): 591–596.

Suter SL, Nolan JJ, Wallace P, Gumbiner B, Olefsky JM. Metabolic effects of new oral hypoglycemic agent CS-045 in NIDDM subjects. *Diabetes Care* 1992; **15**(2): 193–203.

Tachibana K, Tachibana S. Transdermal delivery of insulin by ultrasonic vibrations. *J Pharm Pharmacol* 1991; **43**: 270–271.

Temple MY, Bar-Or O, Riddell MC. The reliability and repeatability of the blood glucose response to prolonged exercise in adolescent boys with IDDM. *Diabetes Care* 1995; **18**(3): 326–332.

Thompson RG, Pearson L, Kolterman OG. Effects of 4 weeks' administration of pramlintide, a human amylin analogue, on glycaemia control in patients with IDDM: effects on plasma glucose profiles and serum fructosamine concentrations. *Diabetologia* 1997a; **40**(11): 1278–1285.

Thompson RG, Pearson L, Schoenfeld SL, Kolterman OG. Pramlintide, a synthetic analog of human amylin, improves the metabolic profile of patients with type 2 diabetes using insulin. The Pramlintide in Type 2 Diabetes Group. *Diabetes Care* 1998; **21**(6): 987–993.

Thompson RG, Peterson J, Gottlieb A, Mullane J. Effects of pramlintide, an analog of human amylin, on plasma glucose profiles in patients with IDDM: results of a multicenter trial. *Diabetes* 1997b; **46**(4): 632–636.

Torlone E, Fanelli C, Rambotti AM, Kassi G, Modarelli G, DiVincenzo A, Epifano L, Ciofetta M, Pampanelli S, Brunetti P, et al. Pharmacokinetics, pharmacodynamics, and glucose counterregulation following subcutaneous injection of the monomeric insulin analogue [Lys(B28), Pro (B29)] in IDDM. *Diabetologia* 1994; **37**: 713–720.

UKPDS Group. Effect of intensive blood-glucose control with metformin on complications in overweight patients with type 2 diabetes (UKPDS 34). *Lancet* 1998c; **352**: 854–865.

UKPDS Group. Intensive blood glucose control with sulphonylureas or insulin compared with conventional treatment and risk of complications in patients with type 2 diabetes (UKPDS 33). *Lancet* 1998a; **352**: 837–853.

UKPDS Group. United Kingdom Prospective Diabetes Study 24: a 6-year, randomized, controlled trial comparing sulfonylurea, insulin, and metformin therapy in patients with newly diagnosed type 2 diabetes that could not be controlled with diet therapy. *Ann Intern Med* 1998b; **128**(3): 165–175.

University Group Diabetes Program. A study of the effects of hypoglycemic agents on vascular complications in patients with adult-onset diabetes. I. Design, methods, and baseline results. *Diabetes* 1970; **19**(Suppl 2): 747–783.

Valensi P, Zirinis P, Nicolas P, Perret G, Sandre-Banon D, Attali JR. Effect of insulin concentration on bioavailability during nasal spray administration. *Pathol Biol (Paris)* 1996; **44**(4): 235–240.

Vannasaeng S, Ploybutr S, Nitiyanant W, Peerapatdit T, Vichayanrat A. Effects of alpha-glucosidase inhibitor (acarbose) combined with sulfonylurea or sulfonylurea and metformin in treatment of non-insulin-dependent diabetes mellitus. *J Med Assoc Thai* 1995; **78**(11): 578–585.

van Staa T, Abenhaim L, Monette J. Rates of hypoglycemia in users of sulfonylureas. *J Clin Epidemiol* 1997; **50**(6): 735–741.

Vignati L, Anderson JH Jr, Iversen PW. Efficacy of insulin lispro in combination with NPH human insulin twice per day in patients with insulin-dependent or non-insulin-dependent diabetes mellitus. Multicenter Insulin Lispro Study Group. *Clin Ther* 1997; **19**(6): 1408–1421.

Wang C, Chan V, Yeung RT. Treatment of acromegaly with bromocriptine. *Aust NZ J Med* 1979; **9**(3): 225–232.

Wilholm BE, Myrhed M. Metformin-associated lactic acidosis in Sweden 1977-1991. *Eur J Clin Pharmacol* 1993; **44**(6): 589–591.

Williams KV, Mullen ML, Kelley DE, Wing RR. The effect of short periods of caloric restriction on weight loss and glycemic control in type 2 diabetes. *Diabetes Care* 1998; **21**(1): 2–8.

Wishart JM, Horowitz M, Morris HA, Jones KL, Nauck MA. Relation between gastric emptying of glucose and plasma concentrations of glucagon-like peptide-1. *Peptides* 1998; **19**(6): 1049–1053.

Wolffenbuttel BH, Nijst L, Sels JP, Menheere PP, Muller PG, Kruseman AC. Effects of a new oral hypoglycemic agent, repaglinide, on metabolic control in sulphonylurea-treated patients with NIDDM. *Eur J Clin Pharmacol* 1993; **45**(2): 113–116.

Wredling R, Liu D, Lins PE, Adamson U. Variation of insulin absorption during subcutaneous and peritoneal infusion in insulin-dependent diabetic patients with unsatisfactory long-term glycemic response to continuous subcutaneous insulin infusion. *Diabet Metab* 1991; **17**(5): 456–459.

Würsch P, Pi-Sunyer FX. The role of viscous soluble fiber in the metabolic control of diabetes. A review with special emphasis on cereals rich in β-glucan. *Diabetes Care* 1997; **20**(11):1774–1780.

Yamamoto A, Umemori S, Muranishi S. Absorption enhancement of intrapulmonary administered insulin by various absorption enhancers and protease inhibitors in rats. *J Pharm Pharmacol* 1994; **46**(1): 14–18.

Yamasaki Y, Kawamori R, Wasada T, Sato A, Omori Y, Eguchi H, Tominaga M, Sasaki H, Ikeda M, Kubota M, et al. Pioglitazone (AD-4833) ameliorates insulin resistance in patients with NIDDM. AD-4833 Glucose Clamp Study Group, Japan. *Tohoku J Exp Med* 1997; **183**(3): 173–183.

Yeater RA, Ullrich IH, Maxwell LP, Goetsch VL. Coronary risk factors in type II diabetes: response to low intensity aerobic exercise. *W V Med J* 1990; **86**(7): 287–290.

Zinman B, Tildesley H, Chiasson JL, Tsui E, Strack T. Insulin lispro in CSII: results of a double-blind crossover study. *Diabetes* 1997; **46**(3): 440–443.

Ziv E, Kidron M, Raz I, Krausz M, Blatt Y, Rotman A, Bar-On H. Oral administration of insulin in solid form to non-diabetic and diabetic dogs. *J Pharm Sci* 1994; **83**(6): 792–794.

5

ASSESSMENT OF GLYCEMIC
CONTROL

The importance of monitoring glycemic control in diabetic patients is well established. However, the selection of an optimal assessment is dependent upon several factors, including the time frame of interest, type of diabetes, current antidiabetic therapy, and cost. In addition, monitoring for the purpose of optimizing an individual treatment regimen must be distinguished from monitoring overall glycemic control in the clinical trial setting. Outcome measures for clinical trials of antidiabetic therapies are discussed in Chapter 9.

URINE GLUCOSE

Urine glucose concentrations reflect blood glucose levels during the period of urine production. Thus, the concentration is an average that is "integrated" over time. As the renal threshold for glucose is approximately 180 mg/dL, a negative urine test indicates that the mean blood glucose concentration was below this threshold during the interval prior to collection. This test is simple and inexpensive to perform, and is thus the most commonly used method worldwide to assess glycemic control. However, the results of the urine test can only provide approximate information about glucose levels above the renal threshold, and thus cannot distinguish between hypoglycemia, euglycemia, and mild to moderate hyperglycemia (Goldstein & Little, 1997). This drawback can be a particular disadvantage in patients receiving insulin therapy, as the risk for hypoglycemia should be carefully monitored in this population.

SELF-MONITORING OF BLOOD GLUCOSE

Direct assessment of capillary blood glucose can provide a reasonably accurate evaluation of day-to-day glycemic control, and may be performed by patients with the use of self-monitoring devices. Although there is conflicting evidence as to whether self-monitoring of blood glucose enhances metabolic control (Oki et al., 1997; Ziegher et al., 1993; Schiffrin & Belmonte, 1982), the DCCT and other controlled trials have generally implemented self-monitoring as part of the therapeutic intervention (de Alva & Jervell, 1997; Wang et al., 1993; DCCT Research Group, 1993; Ohkubo et al., 1995). In general, the benefits of self-monitoring appear to be greatest for patients receiving insulin therapy, in whom frequent adjustments in treatment may be necessary. Moreover, the capacity to detect asymptomatic hypoglycemia with self-monitoring represents a significant advantage over urine testing (Cox et al., 1994). The most prevalent problem associated with this methodology is the collection of inaccurate results as a result of patient error, highlighting the importance of appropriate training (Campbell et al., 1992).

GLYCATED HEMOGLOBIN (HBA$_{1C}$)

Glycated hemoglobin (HbA$_{1c}$) is the most commonly used assessment of longer-term glycemic control. As the rate of HbA$_{1c}$ formation is directly proportional to the level of circulating glucose, HbA$_{1c}$ levels provide a reflection of mean glycemia over the previous 120 days (the average erythrocyte life span). However, it should be noted that HbA$_{1c}$ values are known to be more affected by recent glycemic exposure (within one month) than by more distant exposures (2–4 months prior to assessment; Tahara & Shima, 1993). The clinical significance of HbA$_{1c}$ evaluation was conclusively proven in the DCCT, which demonstrated that glycemic control based on this measure was associated with a dramatic reduction in microvascular complications (DCCT Research Group, 1993). Thus, HbA$_{1c}$ is considered to be the gold standard for the evaluation of glycemic control in diabetic patients.

GLYCATED SERUM PROTEIN

Levels of glycated serum protein also provide an index of average glycemic control over an extended period of time. However, glycated protein assessments reflect a shorter time interval than HbA$_{1c}$, as the turnover of serum albumin (approximately 15–20 days) is much more rapid than for hemoglobin. An advantage of glycated protein assessments is the relatively low expense and time required for analysis; however, the clinical utility of these measures has not been established.

Several measures of glycated protein have been used in the evaluation of long-term glycemic control, including total glycated serum protein, glycated serum albumin, and the fructosamine assay. The fructosamine assay utilizes the ability of glycated protein to act as a reducing agent in an alkaline solution, and has demonstrated comparable results to evaluations of total glycated serum protein and glycated serum albumin (Seng & Staley, 1986; Johnson et al., 1987). However, as significant differences have been observed between results obtained with fructosamine and HbA$_{1c}$, these measures cannot be considered interchangeable (Shield et al., 1994; Fisken et al., 1990). Assessment of glycated protein may be indicated in cases where frequent monitoring is necessary, as in gestational diabetes, or for patients with hemoglobinopathies or reduced erythrocyte survival (Goldstein & Little, 1997).

CONCLUSIONS

Monitoring glycemic control is an important aspect of achieving therapeutic goals. As HbA$_{1c}$ levels have been shown to predict the risk of microvascular complications, this measure has direct clinical significance for patients with diabetes. In addition, short-term assessments such as the self-monitoring of blood glucose can enhance the safety of hypoglycemic therapies, and assist in the individualization of dosing regimens.

References

Campbell LV, Ashwell SM, Borkman M, Chisholm DJ. White coat hyperglycemia: disparity between diabetes clinic and home blood glucose concentrations. *BMJ* 1992; **305**: 1194–1196.

Cox DJ, Kovatchev BP, Julian DM, Gonder-Frederick LA, Polonsky WH, Schlundt DG, Clarke WL. Frequency of severe hypoglycemia in insulin-dependent diabetes mellitus can be predicted from self-monitoring blood glucose data. *J Clin Endocrinol Metab* 1994; **79**(6): 1659–1662.

de Alva M, Jervell J. Self-monitoring improves quality of life and prognosis of people with diabetes [letter]. *BMJ* 1997; **315**: 184–185.

DCCT Research Group. The effect of intensive treatment of diabetes on the development and progression of long-term complications in insulin-dependent diabetes mellitus. *N Engl J Med* 1993; **329**(14): 977–986.

Fisken RA, Chan AW, Hanlon A, Mac Farlane IA, Longitudinal changes in serum fructosamine do not parallel those in glycated haemoglobin in young adults with insulin-dependent diabetes. *Clin Chim Acta* 1990; **191**: 79–86.

Goldstein DE, Little RR. Monitoring glycemia in diabetes. Short-term assessment. *Endocrinol Metab Clin North Am* 1997; **26**(3): 475–486.

Johnson RN, Metcalf PA, Baker JR. Relationship between albumin and fructosamine in diabetic and non-diabetic sera. *Clin Chem Acta* 1987; **164**: 151–162.

Ohkubo Y, Kishikawa H, Araki E, Miyata T, Isami S, Motoyoshi S, Kojima Y. Furuyoshi N, Shichiri M. Intensive insulin treatment prevents the progression of diabetic microvascular complications in Japanese patents with non-insulin-dependent diabetes mellitus: a randomized prospective 6-year study. *Diabetes Res Clin Pract* 1995; **28**(2): 103–117.

Oki JC, Flora DL, Isley WL. Frequency and impact of SMBG on glycemic control in patients with NIDDM in an urban teaching hospital clinic. *Diabetes Educ* 1997; **23**(4): 419–424.

Schiffrin A, Belmonte, MM. Comparison between continuous subcutaneous insulin infusion and multiple injections of insulin. A one-year prospective study. *Diabetes* 1982; **31**(3): 255–264.

Seng LY, Staley MJ. Plasma fructosamine is a measure of all glycated proteins. *Clin Chem* 1986; **32**: 560.

Shield JP, Poyser K, Hunt L, Pencock CA. Fructosamine and glycated hemoglobin in the assessment of long-term glycaemic control in diabetes. *Arch Dis Child* 1994; **71**(5): 443–445.

Tahara Y, Shima Y. The response of GHb to stepwise plasma glucose change over time in diabetic patients [letter]. *Diabetes Care* 1993; **16**: 1313–1314.

Wang PH, Lau J, Chalmers TC. Meta-analysis of effects of intensive blood glucose control on late complications of type I diabetes. *Lancet* 1993; **341**(8856): 1306–1309.

Ziegher O, Kolopp M, Louis J, Musse JP, Patris A, Debry G, Drouin P. Self-monitoring of blood glucose and insulin dose alteration in type 1 diabetes mellitus. *Diabetes Res Clin Pract* 1993; **21**(1): 51–59.

6

CURRENT TREATMENT STRATEGIES TO PREVENT DIABETIC COMPLICATIONS

The development of compounds to directly prevent or treat diabetic complications has the potential to fundamentally change therapeutic strategies for this disease. The progression of micro- and macrovascular complications occurs over the course of several years, suggesting that an adequate window exists for effective therapeutic intervention. Such strategies could expand the therapeutic options for diabetic patients beyond the maintenance of strict glycemic control.

AMINOGUANIDINES AND OTHER ANTI-GLYCATION COMPOUNDS

The development of microangiopathy, macroangiopathy, and associated complications in diabetic patients has been linked to elevated levels of advanced glycation end products (AGEs; Kahaly et al., 1997; Beisswenger et al., 1995), which are formed through the chemical modification of macromolecules by high levels of glucose. These structures are produced via the creation of Schiff bases, followed by a conversion to Amadori products and, finally, AGEs. They are present in increased concentrations in the serum, retina, kidney, and nerve of diabetic patients (Yamaguchi et al., 1998; Ono et al., 1998; Sugimoto et al., 1997; Makita et al., 1991), and have been shown to induce glomerulosclerosis, albuminuria, and vascular dysfunction in normal animals following exogenous administration (Vlassara et al., 1994; Vlassara et al., 1992). It has been postulated that AGEs may promote angiopathies through attachment to and accumulation in the vasculature and the overproduction of reactive oxygen species and oxidative stress (Makita et al., 1996; Brownlee, 1995; Wautier et al., 1994). Thus, a principal strategy for the prevention of complications is the development of compounds that inhibit the formation or activity of AGEs.

Aminoguanidine is the most extensively studied anti-glycation compound, and is currently under clinical investigation for the prevention and treatment of diabetic complications. Aminoguanidine prevents the conversion of Amadori products to AGEs, thus reducing accumulation in the vasculature. In studies with diabetic animals, aminoguanidine administration prevented optic nerve degeneration, renal pathology, and reductions in nerve conduction velocity, indicating potential benefits in the treatment of microangiopathy (Inoue et al, 1998; Miyauchi et al., 1996; Soulis-Liparota et al., 1991). Other evidence suggests that aminoguanidine may also attenuate macrovascular pathology (Corman et al., 1998; Panagiotopoulos et al., 1998). Initial human studies have reported that aminoguanidine reduces hemoglobin AGE levels and plasma LDL cholesterol in diabetic patients (Bucala et al., 1994; Makita et al., 1992). Further clinical trials are underway to evaluate the efficacy of aminoguanidines in the prevention and treatment of diabetic nephropathy and other complications (Skolnick, 1997).

An alternative approach to the prevention of diabetic complications mediated by AGEs is to interfere with their activity at the receptor level. Although AGEs are a heterogeneous group of molecules with several binding sites, one particular site appears to be relevant to the development of microangiopathy (Yan et al., 1997). Expression of the receptor for AGE, or RAGE, appears to be elevated in pathological states including diabetic nephropathy, retinopathy, and neuropathy (Yan et al., 1997; Bierhaus et al., 1996). In the presence of high levels of AGEs, RAGE is thought to contribute to the development of angiopathy through the enhancement of oxidative stress, vascular permeability, and inflammatory cell dysfunction (Wautier et al., 1994; Schmidt et al., 1994). In a preclinical trial, exogenous administration of a soluble form of RAGE resulted in competitive blockade of the receptor and the inhibition of AGE-mediated vascular hyperpermeability in rats (Wautier et al., 1996). However, the effects of soluble RAGE in humans are not yet known, and clinical studies are awaited.

Other approaches targeting AGEs are also under consideration. For example, "crosslink breakers" have demonstrated the ability to cleave existing AGE-derived protein crosslinks *in vitro* and *in vivo*, and to reduce arterial wall stiffness in diabetic mice (Wolffenbuttel et al., 1998). In addition, antioxidants such as vitamin E are also being evaluated for their protective effects against AGE-mediated endothelial damage in diabetic retinopathy (Skolnick, 1997).

ALDOSE REDUCTASE INHIBITORS

Concentrations of aldose reductase are increased in diabetic patients with complications, such as retinopathy and neuropathy, in comparison to patients without complications (Nishimura et al., 1997; Ito et al., 1997; Dent et al., 1991). High circulating levels of glucose have been shown to increase flux through the aldose reductase (or polyol) pathway, resulting in increased transformation of glucose to sorbitol and fructose. As these polyols are not readily permeable to cell membranes, intracellular accumulation can develop, resulting in a reduction of myo-inositol uptake in nerve tissues. These conditions can lead to alterations in nerve conduction and other metabolic consequences, eventually culminating in basement membrane thickening and a reduction of capillary integrity (Tsai & Burnakis, 1993).

Early clinical studies with aldose reductase inhibitors such as ponalrestat did not find long-term benefits in diabetic patients with neuropathy (Florkowski et al., 1991; Ziegler et al., 1991). However, it has been suggested that methodological limitations may have affected the outcomes of these studies (Krans, 1992). For example, many initial studies of aldose reductase inhibitors employed outcome measures that were difficult to interpret, or included patients that varied widely in disease severity. Tolrestat, which was approved for clinical use in several countries, demonstrated more positive results in clinical studies. For example, tolrestat therapy was reported to improve measures of autonomic neuropathy (Didangelos et al., 1998; Fabiani et al., 1995), peripheral neuropathy (Giugliano et al., 1995; Boulton et al., 1990), and retinopathy (van Gerven et al., 1994) in diabetic patients. Moreover, withdrawal of tolrestat in patients that had been treated for an average of 4.2 years was associated with a significant worsening of peripheral neuropathy in comparison to patients who continued to receive the drug (Santiago et al., 1993).

However, reports of liver dysfunction and limited efficacy led to the withdrawal of tolrestat from the market by the manufacturer in 1996 (Foppiano & Lombardo, 1997). Other aldose reductase inhibitors are currently in development that appear to have superior efficacy to tolrestat without its adverse hepatic effects. Thus, aldose reductase inhibitors remain a potential option for the treatment of diabetic complications.

ANGIOTENSIN-CONVERTING ENZYME INHIBITORS

Hypertension is implicated in the development of both micro- and macrovascular complications in diabetic patients. Although the mechanisms underlying this association are unclear, increased vascular pressure may increase the damage to vessel walls, contributing to atherosclerosis and reduced capillary integrity. For example, increased glomerular pressure is associated with the progression of basement membrane thickening and the emergence of overt nephropathy in diabetic patients, indicating that antihypertensive therapy may be an effective strategy to treat or prevent this complication.

Angiotensin-converting enzyme inhibitors (ACE inhibitors) have been employed successfully in the treatment of hypertension in diabetic patients. Agents of this class regulate the balance between the vasoconstrictive actions of angiotensin II and the vasodilatory properties of bradykinin (Brown & Vaughan, 1998). ACE inhibitors such as lisinopril and ramipril have been shown to reduce blood pressure, improve renal dysfunction, and delay the development of end-stage renal failure in hypertensive diabetic patients (Yokoyama et al., 1997; The GISEN Group, 1997). However, evidence suggests that these compounds may have renoprotective effects beyond their impact on hypertension, as ACE inhibitor therapy has also been shown to slow the progression of renal disease in normotensive diabetic patients with microalbuminuria (The Euclid Study Group, 1997; Laffel et al., 1995). In addition, although most studies of ACE inhibitors in diabetes have evaluated effects on nephropathy, results of the recent EUCLID study suggest that lisinopril may also reduce the incidence of retinopathy in normotensive patients with type 1 diabetes (Chaturvedi et al., 1998). Additional clinical studies will be necessary to confirm this finding.

There has been some debate as to the superiority of ACE inhibitors over other types of antihypertensives in the treatment and prevention of diabetic nephropathy. While several studies have indicated that ACE inhibitor therapy results in greater improvements in albuminuria and glomerular filtration than other antihypertensive compounds (Guasch et al., 1997; Rossing et al., 1997; Agardh et al., 1996; Hansson, 1995), others have not reported significant differences in efficacy for ACE inhibitors and calcium channel blockers (Donnelly et al., 1996; Velussi et al., 1996; O'Donnell et al., 1993). Moreover, preliminary clinical evidence suggests that combination therapy with ACE inhibitors and calcium channel blockers may be more effective than either agent alone in slowing the progression of diabetic nephropathy (Ritz et al., 1997; Bakris et al., 1992).

However, important differences have begun to emerge between ACE inhibitors and calcium channel blockers in the prevention of cardiovascular events in diabetic patients. Recent results from the Appropriate Blood Pressure Control in Diabetes (ABCD) Trial indicated that treatment with the calcium channel blocker, nisoldipine, was associated with a greater risk of fatal and non-fatal myocardial infarction than treatment with enalapril in hypertensive type 2 diabetic patients (Estacio et al., 1998). In an interim analysis conducted after five years of therapy, a total of 25 patients in the nisoldipine group (n=235) had experienced a myocardial infarction compared to 5 patients in the enalapril group (n=235). These results are supported by the Fosinopril versus Amlodipine Cardiovascular Events Randomized Trial (FACET), which found that hypertensive type 2 diabetic patients receiving fosinopril had a significantly lower risk of the combined outcome of acute myocardial infarction, stroke, or hospitalized angina than patients receiving amlodipine (Tatti et al., 1998). Although no conclusions can be drawn regarding whether these differences are due to deleterious effects with calcium channel blockers or protective effects with ACE inhibitors, these results indicate that ACE inhibitors are preferred for the treatment of diabetic patients with hypertension.

As insulin-sensitizing effects have previously been described with ACE inhibitor therapy, the risk of hypoglycemia in diabetic patients receiving these agents warrants consideration (Valensi et al., 1996; Raccah et al., 1994). In two retrospective case-control studies of diabetic patients, ACE inhibitor therapy was significantly associated with an increased risk of hospital admission for severe hypoglycemia (Morris et al., 1997; Herings et al., 1995). Such effects have not generally been reported for other antihypertensive agents. However, in a later retrospective cohort study, specific antihypertensive therapy did not affect the risk of hypoglycemia in older diabetic patients (Shorr et al., 1997). These results suggest that ACE inhibitor therapy should not be avoided based solely on the risk of hypoglycemic adverse events, but that monitoring in high-risk populations may be warranted.

CARNITINE ACTIVATORS

The development of neuropathy has been linked to reduced levels of L-carnitine and defective fatty acid metabolism in diabetic patients (Ido et al., 1994; De Palo et al., 1981). Carnitine activators, such as acetyl-L-carnitine, promote fatty acid beta-oxidation in the liver, and have been shown to normalize peripheral nerve function and promote nerve regeneration in animal models of diabetes (Soneru et al., 1997; Sima et al., 1996; Lowitt et al., 1995; Morabito et al., 1993). The efficacy of acetyl-L-carnitine in the improvement of nerve conduction velocity *in vivo* appears to be similar to that of the aldose reductase inhibitor, sorbinil (Malone et al., 1996). Reports of controlled clinical studies evaluating the efficacy of acetyl-L-carnitine therapy in diabetic patients with peripheral neuropathy are awaited.

ANTI-ISCHEMICS

A more downstream approach to the treatment of diabetic complications involves insulating cells from vascular disturbances associated with micro- and macroangiopathy. Bimoclomol is an anti-ischemic compound which has demonstrated protective and restorative effects on microvascular function in diabetic rats, potentially through the induction of various heat shock proteins (Vigh et al., 1997; Biro et al., 1997). Due to these promising *in vivo* results, bimoclomol is currently under clinical investigation as a treatment for diabetic complications.

CONCLUSIONS

Over the past two decades, therapeutic strategies in diabetes have expanded beyond the improvement of glycemic control to the prevention and treatment of its associated complications. It may be several years before the outcomes of large clinical trials evaluating these approaches are known. However, the work that has already been accomplished in this area provides a foundation for the development of therapeutic options previously unavailable to diabetic patients.

References

Agardh CD, Garcia-Puig J, Charbonnel B, Angelkort B, Barnett AH. Greater reduction of urinary albumin excretion in hypertensive type II diabetic patients with incipient nephropathy by lisinopril than by nifedipine. *J Hum Hypertens* 1996; **10**(3): 185–192.

Bakris GL, Barnhill BW, Sadler R. Treatment of arterial hypertension in diabetic humans: importance of therapeutic selection. *Kidney Int* 1992; **41**: 912–919.

Beisswenger PJ, Makita Z, Curphey TJ, Moore LL, Jean S, Brinck-Johnsen T, Bucala R, Vlassara H. Formation of immunochemical advanced glycosylation end products precedes and correlates with early manifestations of renal and retinal disease in diabetes. *Diabetes* 1995; **44**(7): 824–829.

Bierhaus A, Ritz E, Nawroth PP. Expression of receptors for advanced glycation end-products in occlusive vascular and renal disease. *Nephrol Dial Transplant* 1996; **11**(Suppl 5): 87–90.

Biro K, Jednakovits A, Kukorelli T, Hegedus E, Koranyi L. Bimoclomol (BRLP-42) ameliorates peripheral neuropathy in streptozotocin-induced diabetic rats. *Brain Res Bull* 1997; **44**(3): 259–263.

Boulton AJ, Levin S, Comstock J. A multicentre trial of the aldose-reductase inhibitor, tolrestat, in patients with symptomatic diabetic neuropathy. *Diabetologia* 1990; **33**(7): 431–437.

Brown NJ, Vaughan DE. Angiotensin-converting enzyme inhibitors. *Circulation* 1998; **97**(14): 1411–1420.

Brownlee M. The pathological implications of protein glycation. *Clin Invest Med* 1995; **18**(4): 275–281.

Bucala R, Makita Z, Vega G, Grundy S, Koschinsky T, Cerami A, Vlassara H. Modification of low density lipoprotein by advanced glycation end products contributes to the dyslipidemia of diabetes and renal insufficiency. *Proc Natl Acad Sci* 1994; **91**(20): 9441–9445.

Chaturvedi N, Sjolie AK, Stephenson JM, Abrahamian H, Keipes M, Castellarin A, Rogulja-Pepeonik Z, Fuller JH. Effect of lisinopril on progression of retinopathy in normotensive people with type 1 diabetes. The EUCLID Study Group. EURODIAB Controlled Trial of Lisinopril in Insulin-Dependent Diabetes Mellitus. *Lancet* 1998; **351**(9095): 28–31.

Corman B, Duriez M, Poitevin P, Heudes D, Bruneval P, Tedgui A, Levy BI. Aminoguanidine prevents age-related arterial stiffening and cardiac hypertrophy. *Proc Natl Acad Sci USA* 1998; **95**(3): 1301–1306.

Dent MT, Tebbs SE, Gonzalez AM, Ward JD, Wilson RM. Neutrophil aldose reductase activity and its association with established diabetic microvascular complications. *Diabet Med* 1991; **8**(5): 439–442.

De Palo E, Gatti R, Sicolo N, Padovan D, Vettor R, Federspil G. Plasma and urine free L-carnitine in human diabetes mellitus. *Acta Diabetol Lat* 1981; **18**(1): 91–95.

Didangelos TP, Karamitsos DT, Athyros VG, Kourtoglou GI. Effect of aldose reductase inhibition on cardiovascular reflex tests in patients with definite diabetic autonomic neuropathy over a period of 2 years. *J Diabetes Complications* 1998; **12**(4): 201–207.

Donnelly R, Molyneaux LM, Willey KA, Yue D. Comparative effects of indapamide and captopril on blood pressure and albumin excretion rate in diabetic microalbuminuria. *Am J Cardiol* 1996; **77**(6): 26B–30B.

Estacio RO, Jeffers BW, Hiatt WR, Biggerstaff SL, Gifford N, Schrier RW. The effect of nisoldipine as compared with enalapril on cardiovascular outcomes in patients with non-insulin-dependent diabetes and hypertension. *N Engl J Med* 1998; **338**(10): 645–652.

The Euclid Study Group. Randomised placebo-controlled trial of lisinopril in normotensive patents with insulin-dependent diabetes and normoalbuminuria or microalbuminuria. *Lancet* 1997; **349**(9068): 1787–1792.

Fabiani F, De Vincentis N, Staffilano A. Effect of tolrestat on oesophageal transit time and cholescystic motility in type 2 diabetic patients with asymptomatic diabetic neuropathy. *Diabet Metab* 1995; **21**(5): 360–364.

Florkowski C, Rowe B, Nightingale S, Harvey T, Barnett A. Clinical and neurophysiological studies of the aldose reductase inhibitor, ponalrestat, in chronic symptomatic diabetic peripheral neuropathy. *Diabetes* 1991; **40**: 129–133.

Foppiano M, Lombardo G. Worldwide pharmacovigilance systems and tolrestat withdrawal. *Lancet* 1997; **349**: 399–400.

The GISEN Group. Randomised placebo-controlled trial of effect of ramipril on decline in glomerular filtration rate and risk of terminal renal failure in proteinuric, non-diabetic nephropathy. *Lancet* 1997; **349**(9069): 1857–1863.

Giugliano D, Acampora R, Marfella R, Di Maro G, De Rosa N, Misso L, Ceriello A,

Quatraro A, D'Onofrio F. Tolrestat in the primary prevention of diabetic neuropathy. *Diabetes Care* 1995; **18**(4): 536–541.

Guasch A, Parham M, Zayas CF, Campbell O, Nzerue C, Macon E. Contrasting effects of calcium channel blockade versus converting enzyme inhibition on proteinuria in African Americans with non-insulin-dependent diabetes mellitus and nephropathy. *J Am Soc Nephrol* 1997; **8**(5): 793–798.

Hansson L. Effects of angiotensin-converting enzyme inhibition versus conventional antihypertensive therapy on the glomerular filtration rate. *Cardiology* 1995; **86**(Suppl 1): 30–33.

Herings RM, de Boer A, Stricker BH, Leufkens HG, Porsius A. Hypoglycemia associated with use of inhibitors of angiotensin converting enzyme. *Lancet* 1995; **345**(8959): 1195–1198.

Ido Y, McHowat J, Chang KC, Arrigoni-Martelli E, Orfalian Z, Kilo C, Corr PB, Williamson JR. Neural dysfunction and metabolic imbalances in diabetic rats. Prevention by acetyl-l-carnitine. *Diabetes* 1994; **43**(12): 1469–1477.

Ino-ue M, Ohgiya N, Yamamoto M. Effect of aminoguanidine on optic nerve involvement in experimental diabetic rats. *Brain Res* 1998; **800**(2): 319–322.

Ito T, Nishimura C, Takahashi Y, Saito T, Omori Y. The level of erythrocyte aldose reductase: a risk factor for diabetic neuropathy? *Diabetes Res Clin Pract* 1997; **36**(3): 161–167.

Kahaly G, Hansen C, Otto E, Forster G, Beyer J, Hommel G. Diabetic microangiopathy and urinary glycosaminoglycans. *Exp Clin Endocrinol Diabetes* 1997; **105**(3): 145–151.

Krans HM. Recent clinical experience with aldose reductase inhibitors. *J Diabetes Complications* 1992; **6**: 39–44.

Laffel LM, McGill JB, Gans DJ. The beneficial effect of angiotensin-converting enzyme inhibition with captopril on diabetic nephropathy in normotensive IDDM patients with microalbuminuria. North American Microalbuminuria Study Group. *Am J Med* 1995; **99**(5): 497–504.

Lowitt S, Malone JI, Salem AF, Korthals J, Benford S. Acetyl-l-carnitine corrects the altered peripheral nerve function of experimental diabetes. *Metabolism* 1995; **44**(5): 677–680.

Makita Z, Radoff S, Rayfield EJ, Yang Z, Skolnik E, Delaney V, Friendman EA, Cerami A, Vlassara H. Advanced glycosylation end products in patients with diabetic nephropathy. *N Engl J Med* 1991; **325**(12): 836–842.

Makita Z, Vlassara H, Rayfield E, Cartwright K, Friedman E, Rodby R, Cerami A, Bucala R. Hemoglobin-AGE: a circulating marker of advanced glycosylation. *Science* 1992; **258**(5082): 651–653.

Makita Z, Yanagisawa K, Kuwajima S, Bucala R, Vlassara H, Koike T. The role of advanced glycosylation end-products in the pathogenesis of atherosclerosis. *Nephrol Dial*

Transplant 1996; **11**(Suppl 5): 31–33.

Malone JI, Lowitt S, Salem AF, Miranda C, Korthals JK, Carver J. The effects of acetyl-l-carnitine and sorbinil on peripheral nerve structure, chemistry, and function in experimental diabetes. *Metabolism* 1996; **45**(7): 902–907.

Miyauchi Y, Shikama H, Takasu T, Okayima H, Umeda M, Hirasaki E, Ohata I, Nakayama H, Nakagawa S. Slowing of peripheral motor nerve conduction was ameliorated by aminoguanidine in streptozotocin-induced diabetic rats. *Eur J Endocrinol* 1996; **134**(4): 467–473.

Morabito E, Serafini S, Corsico N, Martelli EA. Acetyl-l-carnitine effect of nerve conduction velocity in streptozotocin-diabetic rats. *Arzneimittelforschung* 1993; **43**(3): 343–346.

Morris AD, Boyle DI, McMahon AD, Pearce H, Evans JM, Newton RW, Jung RT, MacDonald TM. ACE inhibitor use is associated with hospitalization for severe hypoglycemia in patients with diabetes. DARTS/MEMO Collaboration. Diabetes Audit and Research in Tayside, Scotland. Medicines Monitoring Unit. *Diabetes Care* 1997; **20**(9): 1363–1367.

Nishimura C, Hota Y, Gui T, Seko A, Fujimaki T, Ishikawa T, Hayakawa M, Kanai A, Saito T. The level of erythrocyte aldose reductase is associated with the severity of diabetic retinopathy. *Diabetes Res Clin Pract* 1997; **37**(3): 173–177.

O'Donnell MJ, Rowe BR, Lawson N, Horton A, Gyde OH, Barnett AH. Comparison of the effects of an angiotensin converting enzyme inhibitor and a calcium antagonist in hypertensive, macroproteinuric diabetic patients: a randomised double-blind study. *J Hum Hypertens* 1993; **7**(4): 333–339.

Ono Y, Aoki S, Ohnishi K, Yasuda T, Kawano K, Tsukada Y. Increased serum levels of advanced glycation end products in NIDDM patients with diabetic complications [letter]. *Diabetes Care* 1998; **21**(6): 1027.

Panagiotopoulos S, O'Brien RC, Bucala R, Cooper ME, Jerums G. Aminoguanidine has an anti-atherogenic effect in the cholesterol-fed rabbit. *Atherosclerosis* 1998; **136**(1): 125–131.

Raccah D, Pettenuzzo-Mollo M, Provendier O, Boucher L, Cozie JA, Gorlier R, Huin P, Sicard J, Vague P. Comparison of the effects of captopril and nicardipine on insulin sensitivity and thrombotic profile in patients with hypertension and android obesity. CaptISM Study Group. Captopril Insulin Sensitivity Multicenter Study Group. *Am J Hypertens* 1994; **7**(8): 731–738.

Ritz E, Orth SR, Strzelczyk P. Angiotensin converting enzyme inhibitors, calcium channel blockers, and their combination in the treatment of glomerular disease. *J Hypertens Suppl* 1997; **15**(2): S21–S26.

Rossing P, Tarnow L, Boelskifte S, Jensen BR, Nielsen FS, Parving HH. Differences between nisoldipine and lisinopril on glomerular filtration rates and albuminuria in hypertensive IDDM patients with diabetic nephropathy during the first year of treatment.

Diabetes 1997; **46**(3): 481–487.

Santiago JV, Snksen PH, Boulton AJ, Macleod A, Beg M, Bochenek W, Graepel GJ, Gonen B. Withdrawal of the aldose reductase inhibitor tolrestat in patients with diabetic neuropathy: effect on nerve function. The Tolrestat Study Group. *J Diabetes Complications* 1993; **7**(3): 170–178.

Schmidt AM, Hori O, Brett J, Yan SD, Wautier JL, Stern D. Cellular receptors for advanced glycation end products. Implications for induction of oxidative stress and cellular dysfunction in the pathogenesis of vascular lesions. *Arterioscler Thromb* 1994; **14**(10): 1521–1528.

Shorr RI, Ray WA, Daugherty JR, Griffin MR. Antihypertensives and the risk of serious hypoglycemia in older persons using insulin or sulfonylureas. *JAMA* 1997; **278**(1): 40–43.

Sima AA, Ristic H, Merry A, Kamijo M, Lattimer SA, Stevens MJ, Greene DA. Primary preventive and secondary interventionary effects of acetyl-l-carnitine on diabetic neuropathy in the bio-breeding Worcester rat. *J Clin Invest* 1996; **97**(8): 1900–1907.

Skolnick AA. Novel therapies to prevent diabetic retinopathy. *JAMA* 1997; **278**(18): 1480–1481.

Soneru IL, Khan T, Orfalian Z, Abraira C. Acetyl-l-carnitine effects on nerve conduction and glycemic regulation in experimental diabetes. *Endocr Res* 1997; **23**(1–2): 27–36.

Soulis-Liparota T, Cooper M, Papazoglou D, Clarke B, Jerums G. Retardation by aminoguanidine of development of albuminuria, mesangial expansion, and tissue fluorescence in streptozotocin-induced diabetic rat. *Diabetes* 1991; **40**(10): 1328–1334.

Sugimoto K, Nishizawa Y, Horiuchi S, Yagihashi S. Localization in human diabetic peripheral nerve of N(epsilon)-carboxymethyllysine protein adducts, an advanced glycation endproduct. *Diabetologia* 1997; **40**(12): 1380–1387.

Tatti P, Pahor M, Byington RP, Di Mauro P, Guarisco R, Strollo G, Strollo F. Outcome results of the Fosinopril Versus Amlodipine Cardiovascular Events Randomized Trial (FACET) in patients with hypertension and NIDDM. *Diabetes Care* 1998; **21**(4): 597–603.

Tsai SC, Burnakis TG. Aldose reductase inhibitors: an update. *Ann Pharmacother* 1993; **27**: 751–754.

Valensi P, Derobert E, Genthon R, Riou JP. Effect of ramipril on insulin sensitivity in obese patients. Time-course study of glucose infusion rate during euglycemic hyperinsulinemic clamp. *Diabete Metab* 1996; **22**(3): 197–200.

van Gerven JM, Boot JP, Lemkes HH, van Best JA. Effects of aldose reductase inhibition with tolrestat on diabetic retinopathy in a six month double blind trial. *Doc Opthamol* 1994; **87**(4): 355–365.

Velussi M, Brocco E, Frigato F, Zolli M, Muollo B, Maioli M, Carraro A, Tonolo G, Fresu P, Cernigoi AM, et al. Effects of cilazapril and amlodipine on kidney function in hypertensive NIDDM patients. *Diabetes* 1996; **45**(2): 216–222.

Vigh L, Literati PN, Horvath I, Torok Z, Balogh G, Glatz A, Kovacs E, Boros I, Ferdiandy P, Farkas B, et al. Bimoclomol: a nontoxic, hydroxylamine derivative with stress protein-inducing activity and cytoprotective effects. *Nat Med* 1997; **3**(10): 1150–1154.

Vlassara H, Fuh H, Makita Z, Krungkrai S, Cerami A, Bucala R. Exogenous advanced glycosylation end products induce complex vascular dysfunction in normal animals: a model for diabetic and aging populations. *Proc Natl Acad Sci* 1992; **89**(24): 12043–12047.

Vlassara H, Striker LJ, Teichberg S, Fuh H, Li YM, Steffes M. Advanced glycation end products induce glomerular sclerosis and albuminuria in normal rats. *Proc Natl Acad Sci USA* 1994; **91**(24): 11704–11708.

Wautier JL, Wautier MP, Schmidt AM, Anderson GM, Hori O, Zoukourian C, Capron L, Chappey O, Yan SD, Brett J, et al. Advanced glycation end products (AGEs) on the surface of diabetic erythrocytes bind to the vessel wall via a specific receptor inducing oxidant stress in the vasculature: a link between surface-associated AGEs and diabetic complications. *Proc Natl Acad Sci USA* 1994; **91**(16): 7742–7746.

Wautier JL, Zoukourian C, Chappey O, Wautier MP, Guillausseau PJ, Cao R, Hori O, Stern D, Schmidt AM. Receptor-mediated endothelial cell dysfunction in diabetic vaculopathy. Soluble receptor for advanced glycation end products blocks hyperpermeability in diabetic rats. *J Clin Invest* 1996; **97**(1): 238–243.

Wolffenbuttel BH, Boulanger CM, Crijns FR, Huijberts MS, Poitevin P, Swennen GN, Vasan S, Egan JJ, Ulrich P, Cerami A, et al. Breakers of advanced glycation end products restore large artery properties in experimental diabetes. *Proc Natl Acad Sci* 1998; **95**(8): 4630–4634.

Yamaguchi M, Nakamura N, Nakano K, Kitagawa Y, Shigeta H, Hasegawa G, Ienaga K, Nakamura K, Nakazawa Y, Fukui I, et al. Immunochemical quantification of crossline as a fluorescent advanced glycation endproduct in erythrocyte membrane proteins from diabetic patients with or without retinopathy. *Diabet Med* 1998; **15**(6): 458–462.

Yan SD, Stern D, Schmidt AM. What's the RAGE? The receptor for advanced glycation end products (RAGE) and the dark side of glucose. *Eur J Clin Invest* 1997; **27**: 179–181.

Yokoyama H, Tomonaga O, Hirayama M, Ishii A, Takeda M, Babazono T, Ujihara U, Takahashi C, Omori Y. Predictors of the progression of diabetic nephropathy and the beneficial effect of angiotensin-converting enzyme inhibitors in NIDDM patients. *Diabetologia* 1997; **40**(4): 405–411.

Ziegler D, Mayer P, Rathmann W, Gries FA. One-year treatment with the aldose reductase inhibitor, ponalrestat, in diabetic neuropathy. *Diabetes Res Clin Pract* 1991; **14**: 63–74.

7

REVIEW OF ANTIDIABETIC COMPOUNDS DEVELOPED IN THE MODERN ERA

The development of oral anti-hyperglycemic agents revolutionized the treatment of type 2 diabetes, and expanded options for patients formerly dependent upon insulin therapy. From 1994 to 1997, six new compounds and four new drug classes were introduced in the U.S. for the treatment of diabetes (Table 7.1). In addition to providing a greater arsenal of potential treatment strategies, however, the diversity of compounds has also complicated the drug development process as multiple combinations of drugs are now possible, and development programs must take this into account. Moreover, it has become increasingly clear that there are no ideal compounds for the long-term treatment of type 2 diabetes, particularly as monotherapy. Limitations of clinical trials for antidiabetic compounds include difficulties in evaluating the durability of efficacy and long-term safety.

METFORMIN

Metformin (Glucophage®) is a biguanide anti-hyperglycemic agent that reduces hepatic glucose production and enhances insulin sensitivity in peripheral tissues. Although initially introduced in the 1950s, the development of metformin was delayed in the U.S. due to the withdrawal of a related compound, phenformin, from the market in 1977; phenformin was found to be associated with an unacceptable risk of lactic acidosis, and consequently raised questions regarding the safety of other biguanide agents. However, epidemiological data from Canada and Europe, where metformin had been marketed continuously for as many as 30 years, indicated that the risk of this adverse event was significantly lower with metformin than with phenformin, thus opening the door for metformin's development and eventual approval by the FDA in 1994. Differences between phenformin and metformin in structure and biological behavior are listed in Table 7.2.

Several small, controlled clinical trials indicated that metformin was superior to placebo in its capacity to lower blood glucose and HbA_{1c} in patients with type 2 diabetes (Nagi & Yudkin, 1993; Dornan et al., 1991). In addition, comparative studies suggested that metformin was as effective as sulfonylurea therapy, without the drawback of weight gain or hypoglycemia (Campbell et al., 1994; Hermann et al., 1991; Clarke & Campbell, 1977).

Table 7.1 - Antidiabetic compounds recently approved in the U.S.

Antidiabetic Compound	Drug Class
metformin (Glucophage®)	biguanide
acarbose (Precose®)	α-glucosidase inhibitor
miglitol (Glyset®)	α-glucosidase inhibitor
glimepiride (Amaryl®)	sulfonylurea
troglitazone (Rezulin®)	thiazolidinedione
repaglinide (Prandin®)	meglitinide

These results were later confirmed in larger pivotal trials. In a randomized, double-blind, placebo-controlled trial, 289 type 2 diabetic patients were placed on a hypocaloric diet for 8 weeks, followed by treatment with metformin titrated to a maximum dose of 2550 mg/day (n=143) or placebo (n=146) for 29 weeks (DeFronzo et al., 1995). Patients were moderately obese (120–170% of ideal weight), and were inadequately controlled by diet alone. By week 29, fasting plasma glucose levels had decreased by 52 mg/dl relative to baseline in patients receiving metformin and had increased by 6 mg/dl in patients receiving placebo ($p<0.001$ metformin versus placebo); HbA_{1c} was reduced by 1.4% and increased by 0.4%, respectively ($p<0.001$). In addition, cholesterol and triglycerides were significantly lower in the metformin group than in the placebo group at the end of the treatment period.

More recently, results from the UKPDS indicated that metformin monotherapy was similarly effective to sulfonylurea or insulin therapy in reducing HbA_{1c} in newly-diagnosed type 2 diabetic patients treated for six years (UKPDS Group, 1998a). Moreover, intensive glycemic control with metformin was more effective than either sulfonylurea (chlorpropamide/glibenclamide) or insulin therapy in reducing the risk of diabetes-related endpoints, all-cause mortality, and stroke in obese diabetic patients (UKPDS Group, 1998b). Metformin was also associated with less weight gain and a lower occurrence of hypoglycemia than insulin or sulfonylureas in obese patients, suggesting that this compound may be the first-line therapy of choice in this population. However, it should be noted that in the UKPDS, only obese patients were randomized to metformin therapy. Therefore, the long-term outcome of metformin therapy for the general type 2 population remains to be demonstrated.

Metformin has also demonstrated safety and efficacy in combination with other antidiabetic agents. For example, metformin was evaluated alone and in combination with sulfonylurea therapy in a randomized, double-blind trial in which 632 moderately obese type 2 diabetic patients received open-label glibenclamide for 5 weeks, followed by random assignment to metformin, titrated to 2550 mg/day (n=210), maximal dose glibenclamide (n=209), or both (n=213) for 29 weeks (DeFronzo et al., 1995). Significant reductions in fasting plasma glucose (63 mg/dl) and HbA_{1c} (1.7%) were observed in patients receiving combination therapy, while values in the other treatment groups increased (glibenclamide alone) or were

Table 7.2 - Differences between phenformin and metformin.

Characteristic	Phenformin	Metformin
Protonation	at terminal imino group	at central amino group
Structure	cyclical; large, liphophilic, planar side chain	not cyclical; hydrophilic
Effects on cellular function and generation of ATP	interferes with electron transfer, suppresses NADH-linked dehydrogenase activity, reduces ATP:ADP ratio at high concentrations	much weaker effects or no effects at all
Aerobic glucose metabolism	increases in peripheral tissues	does not increase in peripheral tissues
Effects on glucose utilization in muscle	high concentrations reduce glycogen stores; low concentrations produce small increases in glucose oxidation, but if concentration increased to upper therapeutic range or beyond, glucose oxidation recedes and lactate production is increased	increases glycogenesis; increases glucose oxidation, but does not significantly increase lactate production (at therapeutic concentrations or order of magnitude above)
Effects on glucose metabolism by adipose tissue	similar to effect on muscle tissue; balance between aerobic and anaerobic glucose metabolism biased toward aerobic at upper therapeutic range	similar to effect on muscle tissue
Binding to plasma proteins	12–20%	none
Metabolism	about 1/3 hydroxylated in liver to inactive metabolite	not measurably metabolized
Clearance	about 75% cleared in 12 hours, much lower in some individuals	almost 90% cleared in 12 hours
Excretion kinetics	first order	multi-exponential
Maximum excretion rate	4.1 mg/h after 50 mg p.o.	100 mg/h after 1000 mg p.o.
% cleared in 48 hours	>99%; greater inter-individual variability in "normal" clearance	>99%; greater capacity for rapid elimination of excessive load
Correlation of drug's clearance to creatinine clearance	poor	good

reduced only slightly (metformin alone; $p<0.001$ combination therapy versus either monotherapy). Lipid profiles also showed improvement in the metformin and combination therapy groups, but remained unchanged in patients receiving glibenclamide monotherapy.

These results were supported by two additional studies. An open-label, multicenter, general practice trial reported that the addition of 850–2550 mg/day metformin to diet and maximal sulfonylurea therapy in 1823 patients with type 2 diabetes resulted in significant reductions from baseline in postprandial blood glucose (91 mg/dl) and HbA_1 (1.9%) by the 12-week endpoint (Haupt et al., 1991). In another 6-month, double-blind trial of 144 type 2 diabetic patients with primary diet failure, combination therapy with high doses of metformin and glibenclamide resulted in significantly greater reductions from baseline in fasting glucose (99 mg/dl) and HbA_{1c} (2.2%) than either treatment alone (Hermann et al., 1994). Metformin and glibenclamide monotherapy produced approximately equal levels of overall glycemic control (HbA_{1c} reductions from baseline of 0.9% and 1.3%, respectively), although only glibenclamide was associated with weight gain and hyperinsulinemia.

Although metformin also appears to be effective as an adjunctive therapy in type 2 diabetic patients receiving insulin, its potential role in the treatment of this population has not yet been resolved (Robinson et al., 1998; Giugliano et al., 1993). As previous studies have suggested that hyperinsulinemia may contribute to atherosclerosis in diabetic patients, the ability to decrease insulin doses may help to reduce macrovascular complications. The addition of metformin to insulin therapy in type 2 diabetic patients has previously been associated with an improvement in glycemic control, allowing for a reduction in insulin dosage and fasting insulin levels (Giugliano et al., 1993). However, the clinical relevance of these effects has not yet been determined in a clinical trial setting.

Adverse events commonly associated with metformin therapy include gastrointestinal effects such as diarrhea, nausea, and abdominal pain. These events tend to be dose-related and to remit with a reduction in dosage level, continuation of therapy beyond 4–6 weeks, or both. Metformin monotherapy is not associated with weight gain, hyperinsulinemia, or hypoglycemia in diabetic patients, which represent advantages over insulin or sulfonylurea therapy. However, a higher incidence of hypoglycemia has been noted with metformin and sulfonylurea combination therapy than with either therapy alone (DeFronzo et al., 1995). Under these conditions, hypoglycemic episodes have generally been mild and limited to a single occurrence.

Unlike its predecessor, phenformin, metformin is only rarely associated with lactic acidosis, with an estimated mean incidence of 0.03 cases per 1000 patient-years (Bailey & Turner, 1996). More recently, the FDA has published the results of post-marketing surveillance for lactic acidosis since its U.S. approval (Misbin et al., 1998). Due to this potential adverse event, however, metformin is contraindicated in individuals with renal impairment, liver disease, congestive heart failure, or a history of lactic acidosis; reported cases of lactic acidosis with metformin therapy have almost exclusively involved patients with these conditions. The sponsor (Bristol-Myers Squibb) is currently conducting a phase IV study in the U.S. to establish the post-marketing rate of lactic acidosis with metformin (The Pink Sheet, January 26, 1998).

In addition, the association of phenformin with an increased risk of cardiovascular mortality in the University Group Diabetes Program (UGDP; University Group Diabetes Program, 1975) raised concerns that metformin may share this adverse effect. Although the results of the UGDP generated some controversy due to the relatively small sample size, the labeling for metformin includes a warning that excess cardiovascular deaths were observed with phenformin therapy in the UGDP. However, the recent results of the UKPDS have diminished this concern, as metformin therapy was actually associated with a reduced incidence of cardiovascular events in comparison to diet therapy in this study (UKPDS Group, 1998b).

ACARBOSE

Acarbose (Precose®) was the first α-glucosidase inhibitor to be approved for clinical use in the U.S. As acarbose does not enhance insulin secretion or activity, it is not associated with the development of hypoglycemia, hyperinsulinemia, or weight gain, all advantages over sulfonylurea therapy. Although its mechanism of action is directed toward the reduction of postprandial hyperglycemia, acarbose also improves overall glycemic control, albeit to a lesser degree than sulfonylurea or biguanide therapy. In addition, the unique mechanism of action of α-glucosidase inhibitor therapy may contribute to its additive effects when used in combination with other antidiabetic treatment regimens.

The efficacy of acarbose in the treatment of type 2 diabetes has been documented in several pivotal clinical trials. In one randomized, double-blind, placebo-controlled trial, 290 type 2 diabetic patients managed on dietary therapy alone received placebo or acarbose at doses of 100, 200, or 300 mg tid for 16 weeks (Coniff et al., 1995a). At endpoint, mean HbA_{1c} levels were significantly reduced by 0.78%, 0.73%, and 1.1% relative to placebo in patients receiving acarbose 100, 200, and 300 mg tid, respectively. In addition, patients treated with acarbose demonstrated significant reductions from baseline in fasting plasma glucose at all three dose levels (range, 7–19 mg/dl), in comparison to an increase of 20 mg/dl in the placebo group. Postprandial plasma glucose reductions of 43, 53, and 98 mg/dl were also observed at doses of 100, 200, and 300 mg tid, respectively, while an increase of 32 mg/dl was seen in placebo-treated patients.

Another major, long-term, placebo-controlled trial of acarbose was conducted in 212 obese patients with type 2 diabetes (Coniff et al., 1994). In this study, patients managed on diet therapy alone were randomized to receive placebo or acarbose, titrated from 50 to 300 mg tid, for 24 weeks. In the endpoint analysis, mean HbA_{1c} was reduced by 0.59% in the acarbose group in comparison to the placebo group ($p \leq 0.0001$). Significant reductions relative to placebo were also observed for fasting (16 mg/dl) and postprandial (50 mg/dl) plasma glucose in patients treated with acarbose. For all of these measures, values decreased in patients receiving acarbose and increased in patients receiving placebo.

Another double-blind, placebo-controlled study evaluated the effects of acarbose in 100 newly-diagnosed diabetic patients who had never used antidiabetic agents, and who were poorly controlled by diet (Hanefield et al., 1991). Patients were randomized to receive placebo or acarbose 100 mg tid for 24 weeks. At the end of treatment, a 0.65% reduction in HbA_1 from baseline was observed with acarbose therapy (p=0.003 versus placebo). Fasting blood glucose levels were also reduced by 25 mg/dl from baseline in patients receiving acarbose, a significantly greater reduction than that observed in placebo-treated patients (p=0.007). In addition, acarbose was superior to placebo in achieving postprandial blood glucose control ($p<0.001$). More recently, the results of the Precose Resolution of Optimal

Titration to Enhance Current Therapies (PROTECT) postmarketing trial, conducted in 6142 type 2 diabetic patients, indicated that acarbose may be particularly effective in recently-diagnosed, drug-naive patients (Buse et al., 1998a). In this open-label trial, patients were titrated to a maximum acarbose dose of 100 mg tid, based on tolerability and efficacy. At endpoint, the mean reduction in HbA_{1c} from baseline was 0.66%; however, in a subset of patients who had been diagnosed for less than one year, the mean reduction from baseline was 1.23%. Additional analysis revealed that patients who were untreated at baseline demonstrated greater improvement than those who were receiving sulfonylureas (reduction in HbA_{1c} of 0.97% versus 0.55%, respectively).

More recently, the FDA approved acarbose for use in combination with insulin or metformin in type 2 diabetes. In a multicenter, randomized, double-blind, placebo-controlled trial, 195 type 2 diabetic patients inadequately controlled by diet and insulin therapy were randomized to receive placebo or additional therapy with acarbose, titrated to a maximum of 100 mg tid (Kelley et al., 1998). After 24 weeks of double-blind therapy, patients receiving acarbose demonstrated a significant reduction in mean HbA_{1c} (0.69%) in comparison to patients receiving placebo. A second study of similar design was conducted in 84 type 2 diabetic patients inadequately controlled on diet and metformin therapy (Rosenstock et al., 1998). Patients receiving acarbose (maximum dose of 100 mg tid) in addition to metformin and diet therapy showed an improvement in mean HbA_{1c} of -0.65% in comparison to those receiving placebo. Significant improvements in postprandial plasma glucose and serum triglyceride levels were also associated with acarbose therapy in both studies. Although gastrointestinal side effects were more frequent in the acarbose group, no differences were observed between groups for hypoglycemia or liver transaminase levels.

Acarbose has also demonstrated efficacy in combination with other antidiabetic agents. In a one-year, double-blind, placebo-controlled trial, a total of 354 patients with type 2 diabetes were randomized to receive acarbose (up to 200 mg tid) or placebo in addition to their current antidiabetic treatment regimen (Chiasson et al., 1994). Patients were analyzed in four groups, according to their treatment regimen at the beginning of the study: diet alone (n=77), diet plus metformin (n=83), diet plus sulfonylurea (n=103), or diet plus insulin (n=91). After one year of treatment, significant reductions in HbA_{1c} for patients treated with acarbose were 0.9% in the diet alone group, 0.8% in the metformin group, 0.9% in the sulfonylurea group, and 0.4% in the insulin group, in comparison to placebo. Patients randomized to receive acarbose also demonstrated a significant reduction in fasting plasma glucose in comparison to placebo in the diet (38 mg/dl) and sulfonylurea (25 mg/dl) groups only. Significant changes in postprandial plasma glucose relative to placebo were also observed for all acarbose-treated patients, ranging from -49 mg/dl (insulin group) to -81 mg/dl (diet alone group). A higher occurrence of gastrointestinal symptoms was associated with acarbose than with placebo; however, these events were mostly mild to moderate in intensity. Thus, combination therapy with acarbose provided additional long-term benefits on glycemic control, regardless of the concomitant antidiabetic agent used.

Another double-blind, placebo-controlled study evaluated the efficacy of acarbose, alone and in combination with tolbutamide, in patients with type 2 diabetes (Coniff et al., 1995b). A total of 290 patients managed by diet alone were randomized to receive placebo, acarbose 200 mg tid, tolbutamide, or a combination of both for 24 weeks. At endpoint, all active treatments were superior to placebo in improving glycemic control ($p<0.05$). In addition, combination therapy with acarbose and tolbutamide was more effective than either agent alone, and tolbutamide monotherapy was more effective than acarbose monotherapy. The mean reduction in postprandial plasma glucose from baseline was 85 mg/dl for acarbose plus tolbutamide, 71 mg/dl for tolbutamide, 56 mg/dl for acarbose, and 13 mg/dl for placebo; corresponding changes in HbA_{1c} were -1.3%, -0.9%, -0.5%, and an increase of 0.04%, respectively. By the end of the study, significantly lower mean doses of tolbutamide were reported for patients receiving combination therapy than for patients receiving monotherapy. Both combination therapy and acarbose monotherapy were associated with an increased incidence of gastrointestinal side effects, but were well tolerated overall. Tolbutamide therapy was associated with an increase in weight and hyperinsulinemia, but these effects were not observed with combination therapy. Elevations in transaminase levels occurred in three patients receiving acarbose monotherapy and two patients receiving acarbose plus tolbutamide. All values returned to normal with the cessation of therapy.

Consistent with the local activity of α-glucosidase inhibitors in the intestinal lumen, the most common adverse events observed in clinical trials of acarbose were flatulence, abdominal pain, and diarrhea. These effects were generally dose-related, transient, and mild to moderate in intensity. Acarbose monotherapy has a very low risk of hypoglycemia, but may contribute to an increased risk when combined with other antidiabetic agents. Other systemic effects have also been reported. Elevations in serum transaminase levels have been observed at doses above 300 mg, although these incidents were generally asymptomatic. International postmarketing surveillance of approximately 3 million patient-years of acarbose exposure has documented 62 cases of elevated serum transaminase levels greater than 500 IU/L, 29 of which were associated with jaundice (Physician's Desk Reference, 1999). Most of these cases occurred in patients weighing less than 60 kg, and the abnormalities generally resolved or improved with the discontinuation of therapy. Thus, regular monitoring of serum transaminase levels is recommended every three months during the first year of therapy, followed by periodic testing thereafter; elevations may indicate that discontinuation or dosage reductions are warranted (Yee & Fong, 1996).

MIGLITOL

Miglitol (Glyset®) was the second α-glucosidase inhibitor to be approved in the U.S. for the treatment of diabetes. Although approved in 1996, the manufacturer (Bayer) did not immediately market miglitol, presumably due to its similarity to acarbose, another Bayer compound. Miglitol is metabolically distinct from acarbose in that it is absorbable, although its activity appears to be limited to the intestinal lumen at clinical doses. Like other members of its class, it does not cause hypoglycemia, hyperinsulinemia, or weight gain, but is associated with gastrointestinal adverse events.

The efficacy and safety of miglitol monotherapy have been evaluated in comparison to sulfonylurea treatment in patients with type 2 diabetes previously treated with diet alone. In one double-blind study, 100 patients were randomized to receive miglitol (50 mg tid for 6 weeks followed by 100 mg tid) or maximal dose glibenclamide for 24 weeks (Pagano et al., 1995). At the end of the treatment period, improvements in HbA_{1c} from baseline were observed in patients receiving both miglitol (-0.8%, $p=0.0003$) and glibenclamide (-1.2, $p=0.0001$). Efficacy on this measure did not differ significantly between treatment groups at endpoint, although glibenclamide was associated with a more rapid treatment response. Fasting plasma glucose was also similarly reduced by 16 mg/dl in the miglitol group

(p=0.005) and 20 mg/dl in the glibenclamide group (p=0.007) in comparison to pretreatment values, while a greater improvement in postprandial glucose excursions was observed in patients receiving miglitol (-56 mg/dl versus -36 mg/dl). A similar overall incidence of adverse events was observed in both treatment groups, although miglitol therapy was associated with gastrointestinal events while glibenclamide was associated with asthenia.

The comparative safety and efficacy of miglitol and glibenclamide therapy were also evaluated in a double-blind, placebo-controlled trial conducted in 201 type 2 diabetic patients (Segal et al., 1997). In this study, patients were randomized to receive miglitol (50 mg tid for 4 weeks followed by 100 mg tid), glibenclamide, or placebo for a total of 24 weeks. In comparison to placebo, the mean baseline-adjusted HbA$_{1c}$ was reduced by 0.8% (p=0.002) in patients receiving miglitol, and 1.0% (p=0.0001) in patients receiving glibenclamide. Mean fasting blood glucose also improved relative to baseline in both treatment groups (-10 mg/dl and -14 mg/dl in the miglitol and glibenclamide groups, respectively), in comparison to an increase of 13 mg/dl in the placebo group. Similarly, postprandial blood glucose levels decreased relative to baseline in patients receiving miglitol (31 mg/dl) and glibenclamide (32 mg/dl), while levels increased by 8 mg/dl in patients receiving placebo. As expected, a higher incidence of flatulence and diarrhea was observed with miglitol therapy than with glibenclamide or placebo. However, patients receiving glibenclamide reported more abdominal pain and possible hypoglycemic symptoms than patients in any other group.

As elderly patients may be particularly susceptible to hypoglycemia induced by oral antidiabetic compounds, the long-term efficacy and safety of miglitol were evaluated in comparison to sulfonylurea therapy in elderly type 2 diabetic patients (Johnston et al., 1998). A total of 411 diet-treated patients ages 60 years and older were randomized to receive placebo, 25 mg tid miglitol, 50 mg tid miglitol, or glibenclamide for one year of double-blind therapy. At study endpoint, mean baseline-adjusted HbA$_{1c}$ levels were reduced by 0.49%, 0.40%, and 0.92% in comparison to placebo in the 25 mg tid miglitol, 50 mg tid miglitol, and glibenclamide treatment groups, respectively (p<0.05 versus placebo). A higher incidence of hypoglycemia, weight gain, cardiovascular events, and postprandial hyperinsulinemia was observed in patients receiving glibenclamide than in any other treatment group, while diarrhea and flatulence were more common with miglitol than with glibenclamide or placebo. Thus, miglitol demonstrated a smaller effect on glycemic control but a more favorable safety profile in comparison to sulfonylurea therapy in elderly patients in this study.

Miglitol has also demonstrated safety and efficacy as add-on therapy in patients inadequately treated with sulfonylureas. In a double-blind, placebo-controlled study of 192 type 2 diabetic patients who had received maximal dose sulfonylurea therapy for at least 4 weeks, patients were randomized to receive 50 mg tid miglitol, 100 mg tid miglitol, or placebo for 14 weeks (Johnston et al., 1994). Mean baseline-adjusted reductions in HbA$_{1c}$ were 0.8% and 0.7% relative to placebo (p<0.0001) in the 50 and 100 mg tid miglitol groups, respectively. Improvements in postprandial plasma glucose relative to placebo were -57 mg/dl with 50 mg tid and -64 mg/dl with 100 mg tid, although no significant changes were observed for fasting plasma glucose. Dose-related gastrointestinal adverse events were observed with miglitol therapy, leading to the premature withdrawal of 5% and 15% of patients receiving 50 and 100 mg tid, respectively.

Miglitol may be a useful adjunct to insulin therapy in patients with both type 1 and type 2 diabetes. Early studies found that miglitol reduced postprandial hyperglycemia and insulin requirements in type 1 diabetic patients, without a significant increase in adverse events (Dimitriadis et al., 1986, 1988). A later double-blind study (Mitrakou et al., 1998) evaluated the efficacy and safety of miglitol in type 2 patients receiving insulin therapy. A total of 117 patients were randomized to receive miglitol (50 mg tid for 4 weeks followed by 100 mg tid) or placebo for 24 weeks. A 1.6% reduction in HbA_1 from baseline was observed at endpoint in patients receiving miglitol ($p<0.001$), while levels remained stable in patients receiving placebo. Fasting and postprandial plasma glucose also improved by -25 mg/dl and -74 mg/dl, respectively, in the miglitol group; corresponding changes were -9 mg/dl and -13 mg/dl in the placebo group. Miglitol was associated with gastrointestinal adverse events which resolved with the continuation of therapy.

The adverse event profile of miglitol is similar to that of other α-glucosidase inhibitors, and includes flatulence, diarrhea, and abdominal pain. These events tend to be dose-related and to decrease over time, although they may result in discontinuation of treatment in some patients. It has been suggested that miglitol may be associated with fewer adverse events than acarbose (Segal et al., 1997), although a controlled comparison has not been reported. Miglitol is not associated with hypoglycemia, hyperinsulinemia, weight gain, or elevations in liver enzymes.

GLIMEPIRIDE

Although sulfonylureas remain a cornerstone of treatment for type 2 diabetes, hypoglycemia and weight gain represent two significant drawbacks to this type of therapy. Thus, the search has continued for safer and more effective sulfonylurea compounds and other insulin secretagogues. Glimepiride (Amaryl®) is the latest sulfonylurea compound to be approved for the treatment of type 2 diabetes. Like other sulfonylureas, glimepiride promotes insulin release by binding to membrane receptors on pancreatic β-cells. However, it has a higher rate of association and disassociation from these receptors *in vitro* than glibenclamide, which may contribute to a more rapid onset of action (Müller et al., 1994). In addition, glimepiride does not appear to exert effects on myocardial potassium channels in humans, which suggests a potentially lower liability for adverse cardiovascular effects. Moreover, glimepiride is effective when administered once daily, which may enhance patient convenience and compliance with this therapy (Sonnenberg et al., 1997).

In a double-blind, placebo-controlled, dose-ranging study, 304 type 2 diabetic patients were randomized to receive placebo or glimepiride at doses of 1, 4, or 8 mg once daily for 14 weeks (Goldberg et al., 1996). At the end of the treatment period, changes in HbA_{1c} from baseline, relative to the placebo group, were -1.2%, -1.8%, and -1.9% in patients receiving 1 mg, 4 mg, and 8 mg glimepiride, respectively ($p<0.001$ versus placebo). Median baseline-adjusted reductions in fasting plasma glucose relative to placebo were 43, 70, and 74 mg/dl in the 1 mg, 4 mg, and 8 mg glimepiride groups, respectively, while corresponding reductions in postprandial glucose levels were 63, 92, and 94 mg/dl ($p<0.001$ versus placebo for both measures). Although the 8 mg dose did not appear to confer additional benefits over the 4 mg dose on average, it was particularly effective in patients with a baseline HbA_{1c} of 8% or more. Glimepiride was well tolerated overall, although symptoms of hypoglycemia and weight gain were reported.

In another study, 249 type 2 diabetic patients for whom dietary therapy was inadequate were randomized to receive glimepiride (up to 8 mg) or placebo once daily for a 10-week dose titration period, followed by a 12-week maintenance period (Schade et al., 1998). At endpoint, HbA_{1c} was reduced by 1.4% units, fasting plasma glucose by 46 mg/dl, and postprandial glucose by 72 mg/dl from baseline levels in patients receiving glimepiride, relative to placebo. The overall incidence of adverse events was similar in both groups, and no hypoglycemic episodes were reported.

Glimepiride was compared with glibenclamide in a double-blind, parallel-group titration study in 577 type 2 diabetic patients treated for one year (Dills et al., 1996). Patients who had previously been treated with sulfonylureas or diet alone were randomized to receive glimepiride or glibenclamide, titrated to a dose which achieved a target fasting plasma glucose range of 90–150 mg/dl and a reduction of at least 25 mg/dl from baseline. Similar reductions in HbA_{1c} from baseline were observed in the glimepiride (0.85%) and glibenclamide (0.83%) groups. Fasting plasma glucose also significantly improved in both treatment groups ($p<0.001$ relative to baseline), with reductions of 49 mg/dl and 44 mg/dl in the glimepiride and glibenclamide groups, respectively. A lower incidence of hypoglycemia was reported in patients receiving glimepiride (12%) than in those receiving glibenclamide (17%).

Similar results were reported in another double-blind, randomized, comparative study of glimepiride and glibenclamide (Draeger et al., 1996). In this trial, 1044 patients received glimepiride (titrated to a maximum dose of 8 mg) or glibenclamide (titrated to a maximum dose of 20 mg) for a total of 12 months. Over the treatment period, the mean HbA_{1c} increased slightly from baseline in both treatment groups (0.4% with glimepiride and 0.3% with glibenclamide), as expected for long-term sulfonylurea therapy. Fasting blood glucose also increased from baseline, by 16 mg/dl in glimepiride-treated patients and 9 mg/dl in glibenclamide-treated patients. Differences between treatment groups were not considered clinically significant for either parameter. A slightly lower occurrence of hypoglycemia was reported with glimepiride (11%) than with glibenclamide (14%).

As sulfonylurea therapy is associated with a high rate of secondary failure, patients may require the addition of insulin or other antidiabetic agents to maintain good glycemic control. In a 24-week, randomized, placebo-controlled, double-blind study conducted in 208 patients with secondary failure to sulfonylurea therapy, glimepiride was found to be safe and well tolerated in combination with an evening dose of insulin (Riddle et al., 1998). Although glycemic control was similar at endpoint in patients receiving placebo and insulin and in those receiving glimepiride and insulin (reduction in HbA_{1c} of approximately 2.1%), clinical responses were more rapid with glimepiride combination therapy. There were no reports of severe hypoglycemia with the addition of glimepiride, and patients were able to maintain lower dosages of insulin.

As with any sulfonylurea, the most common adverse event associated with glimepiride therapy is hypoglycemia. Results of comparative trials in the U.S. suggest that glimepiride may be associated with a lower risk of hypoglycemia than glibenclamide or glipizide, particularly during the first few weeks of therapy, although further confirmation of these results will be necessary before any conclusions can be drawn (Schneider & Chaikin, 1997). Like other sulfonylureas, modest weight gain has been reported with glimepiride therapy. In the 14-week study of type 2 diabetic patients who had previously received sulfonylurea therapy, median body weight in the glimepiride group increased by 0.5 and

0.9 kg at doses of 4 and 8 mg, respectively, in comparison to a reduction of 1.8 kg in the placebo group (Goldberg et al., 1996). The 22-week study of type 2 diabetic patients who had not received oral antidiabetic therapy within 6 months prior to the study also noted a weight increase of 1.8 kg in glimepiride-treated patients in comparison to a reduction of 0.7 kg in placebo-treated patients (Schade et al., 1998). In both of these studies, however, weight gain was unaccompanied by adverse alterations in lipid profiles.

Similar to metformin, the results of the UGDP have cast a long shadow on sulfonylurea therapy in general, as it was reported that tolbutamide was associated with an increased risk of cardiovascular mortality in this study (University Group Diabetes Program, 1975). All sulfonylurea compounds, including newer-generation agents such as glimepiride, have carried this information in their labeling. However, the UKPDS did not find an adverse effect of sulfonylurea therapy (i.e., chlorpropamide, glibenclamide, or glipizide) on cardiovascular events after 10 years (UKPDS Group, 1998c). Moreover, glimepiride's lack of activity at potassium channels in the myocardium suggests the possibility of a reduction in whatever adverse cardiovascular effects may result from non-selective sulfonylurea therapies.

TROGLITAZONE

Troglitazone (Rezulin®) was the first member of the thiazolidinedione class of antidiabetic compounds to be approved for clinical use. Although its underlying mechanism of action has not been completely elucidated, troglitazone binds to the peroxisome proliferative activated receptor-γ. This results in the synthesis of a number of proteins that also follow insulin receptor activation. Troglitazone has demonstrated the capacity to enhance the effects of insulin in peripheral tissues and reduce hepatic gluconeogenesis in patients with diabetes (Sparano & Seaton, 1998; Inzucchi et al., 1998).

The efficacy of troglitazone was first demonstrated in combination with insulin therapy, and this was the first indication to be approved. In a study of 350 patients with poorly controlled type 2 diabetes who were receiving insulin therapy, the addition of 200 or 600 mg/day troglitazone resulted in reductions in fasting serum glucose of 35 and 49 mg/dl, respectively, by the 26-week timepoint (Schwartz et al., 1998). Moreover, adjusted mean HbA_{1c} values decreased by 0.8% in the 200 mg/day group and 1.4% in the 600 mg/day group in comparison to placebo ($p<0.001$), despite insulin dose reductions of 11% and 29%, respectively. A higher occurrence of hypoglycemic symptoms was observed in patients receiving troglitazone 600 mg/day (62%) than in those receiving 200 mg/day (45%) or placebo (41%), suggesting that caution is warranted with higher doses in combination therapy. In another double-blind study, 222 patients on insulin therapy received placebo or 200 or 400 mg/day troglitazone for 26 weeks (Buse et al., 1998b). Responders were defined as having at least a 50% reduction in insulin dose and either a 15% reduction in fasting blood glucose or a blood glucose level of less than 140 mg/dl. By endpoint, 22 and 27% of patients were designated responders in the 200 and 400 mg/day groups, respectively, in comparison to only 7% of placebo-treated patients.

Clinical experience with troglitazone monotherapy has demonstrated its beneficial effects on fasting and postprandial glucose levels, but has indicated only modest effects on long-term measures of glycemic control such as HbA_{1c}. In a double-blind, placebo-controlled, dose-ranging trial, 330 type 2 diabetic patients with inadequate glycemic control were randomized to receive placebo or troglitazone at doses of 200–800 mg/day for 12 weeks (Kumar et al., 1996). By the end of the study, fasting serum glucose was reduced by 18–36 mg/dl in patients receiving troglitazone compared to an increase of 27 mg/dl in those receiving placebo. HbA_{1c} levels increased in the placebo group during the treatment period, but remained unchanged in the troglitazone group. Serum triglyceride concentrations were significantly reduced and high density lipoprotein concentrations were increased at doses of 600 and 800 mg/day. Low density lipoprotein increased at doses of 400 and 600 mg/day, but not at 800 mg/day. Another 12-week, double-blind study, in which type 2 diabetic patients poorly controlled by diet alone were randomized to receive 400 mg/day troglitazone (n=136) or placebo (n=126), reported significant ($p<0.001$) reductions in fasting plasma glucose (23 mg/dl) and HbA_{1c} (0.5%) in the troglitazone group and no change in the placebo group (Iwamoto et al., 1996a). However, only 45.6% of patients receiving troglitazone were classified as responders (greater than 20% reduction in fasting plasma glucose or 1% reduction in HbA_{1c}) in this study.

A 6-month, double-blind, placebo-controlled trial was conducted in 93 patients with type 2 diabetes who were previously treated with diet alone or had discontinued oral antidiabetic medication (Maggs et al., 1998). Patients were randomized to receive placebo or troglitazone at doses of 100, 200, 400, or 600 mg/day. All doses produced improvements in fasting glucose levels by the end of study in a dose-related fashion. Troglitazone reduced fasting plasma glucose by approximately 20% at 400 and 600 mg/day, with improvements of -22 mg/dl and -45 mg/dl, respectively. However, significant improvements in HbA_{1c} from pretreatment levels were not observed in this study. In a similarly designed study, 402 patients with type 2 diabetes were randomized to receive placebo or troglitazone 100, 200, 400, or 600 mg/day for 6 months (Fonseca et al., 1998). At doses of 400 and 600 mg/day, patients treated with troglitazone demonstrated significant reductions relative to placebo in mean fasting serum glucose (51 and 60 mg/dl, respectively) and HbA_{1c} (0.7% and 1.1%, respectively). A subgroup analysis of patients who were on diet and exercise alone prior to the study revealed that only the 600 mg dose of troglitazone produced significant improvements in glycemic control in this population, suggesting that higher doses of troglitazone monotherapy may be necessary in newly-diagnosed type 2 diabetic patients who have not received previous antidiabetic therapy.

Clinical trial experience with troglitazone and oral sulfonylureas provides a basis for combination therapy. In one study, 291 type 2 diabetic patients poorly controlled by sulfonylurea therapy alone were randomized to receive troglitazone 400 mg/day or placebo as add-on therapy for 12 weeks (Iwamoto et al., 1996b). The addition of troglitazone resulted in significant reductions in fasting plasma glucose (29 mg/dl) and HbA_{1c} (0.7%), while no change was observed with the addition of placebo. Adverse events were comparable between the two treatment groups, although a higher percentage of patients receiving troglitazone had reductions in red blood cell mass and hemoglobin levels. These effects resolved with the cessation of therapy. Similar results were reported in a one-year trial evaluating micronized glibenclamide and troglitazone, alone and in combination, in 552 patients with type 2 diabetes inadequately controlled by maximal sulfonylurea monotherapy (Horton et al., 1998). Patients receiving combination therapy had significantly lower mean serum fasting glucose and HbA_{1c} than those receiving either monotherapy at endpoint; both parameters were reduced with combination therapy and increased with monotherapy. All therapies were well tolerated.

As troglitazone works primarily by enhancing insulin sensitivity, it has also demonstrated the capacity to reduce insulin resistance in non-diabetic individuals with normal or impaired glucose tolerance (Antonucci et al., 1997; Nolan et al., 1994). Based on these results, troglitazone was included in an NIH-sponsored study of therapies aimed at preventing the development of overt type 2 diabetes in high-risk individuals (Bloomgarden, 1997). As mentioned in Chapter 3, the troglitazone arm was prematurely discontinued after concerns developed about the benefit-to-risk relationship of this therapy for prevention. Two other studies of troglitazone in diabetes prevention are still pending: the Troglitazone in the Prevention of Diabetes (TRIPOD) study is underway to evaluate the effect of troglitazone administration in non-diabetic women with prior gestational diabetes (Azen et al., 1998), while a multicenter study sponsored by Warner-Lambert to determine whether troglitazone can delay or prevent the progression of impaired glucose tolerance to type 2 diabetes is planned (Scrip No. 2390, 1998).

Troglitazone was generally well tolerated in clinical trials, with an adverse event profile comparable to placebo. Clinical evidence also suggests that troglitazone can be used in elderly patients with type 2 diabetes (Kumar et al., 1998). As monotherapy, troglitazone is not associated with hypoglycemia, although an increased risk has been observed when it is combined with other antidiabetic agents. Reductions in red blood cells, neutrophil counts, hemoglobin, and hematocrit have been consistently observed in clinical trials, but the magnitudes of the changes were modest. These changes appear to be explained by drug-induced increases in plasma volume (Johnson et al., 1998). As noted in Chapter 4, the adverse cardiovascular effects observed in preclinical studies were not detected in human trials of troglitazone (Ghazzi et al., 1997). However, the same effects on plasma volume and levels of formed blood elements have also been seen in animals. These effects, along with a significant effect on body weight seen in both humans and animals, suggest that troglitazone alters body fluid homeostasis. No mechanism has been identified for what appears to be a unique drug effect.

Weight gain was observed in clinical trials of troglitazone as monotherapy or in combination with sulfonylureas. In one study (Iwamoto et al., 1996a), patients receiving troglitazone monotherapy gained a mean of 0.6 kg while patients receiving placebo lost a mean of 0.4 kg (treatment difference, $p<0.001$). Similar results were reported in a study of troglitazone and sulfonylurea combination therapy (Iwamoto et al., 1996b). A mean weight gain of 0.6 kg was observed in the troglitazone treatment group, in comparison to a mean loss of 0.2 kg in the placebo group (treatment difference, $p<0.001$). In both of these studies, however, total and HDL cholesterol did not change, and triglyceride levels were reduced in patients receiving troglitazone.

The most significant safety concern with troglitazone therapy is its potential to induce liver enzyme abnormalities. In controlled clinical trials, reversible elevations in AST or ALT greater than three times the upper limit of normal were observed in 2.2% of patients receiving troglitazone and 0.6% of patients receiving placebo. Figures from the U.S. database of patients enrolled in troglitazone trials indicate that 20 patients discontinued treatment due to liver function abnormalities, although all occurrences were reversible (Henry, 1997). Soon after the approval of troglitazone's indication for monotherapy, several cases of liver failure were reported. As a result, the sale of troglitazone was voluntarily suspended by the sponsor in the U.K. (Glaxo Wellcome), and the drug labeling was revised in the U.S. to recommend liver enzyme monitoring at the start of therapy, every month during the first 6 months, every 2 months for the remainder of the first year, and periodically thereafter (The Pink Sheet, August 3, 1998; Scrip No. 2357, 1998). As of September, 1998, over 30 cases of troglitazone hepatotoxicity have been reported to the FDA. A revision of the warning label in July of 1998 mandates liver enzyme monitoring for up to 8 months.

As troglitazone has been shown to induce the CYP3A4 enzyme system *in vivo*, it may contribute to drug interactions with other compounds metabolized by this system. Interactions have previously been documented with oral contraceptives and terfenadine. Other drugs that may interact with troglitazone include calcium channel blockers, cisapride, corticosteroids, and cyclosporine (Sparano & Seaton, 1998).

REPAGLINIDE

The approval of repaglinide (Prandin®) by the FDA in 1997 marked the introduction of the meglitinide class of antidiabetic compounds for the treatment of type 2 diabetes. Repaglinide stimulates the release of insulin from pancreatic β-cells. *In vitro* data suggest that the activity of repaglinide is mediated via receptor binding sites distinct from the sulfonylureas (Fuhlendorff et al., 1998). As it is rapidly absorbed and eliminated, it has a fast onset and offset of action, which could more accurately mimic physiologic insulin profiles and reduce the risk of hypoglycemia. In addition, repaglinide is administered with meals, which could provide more flexibility than longer-acting therapies that require the patient to eat at regular intervals.

In an initial double-blind, placebo-controlled study, patients who had not previously been treated with sulfonylureas were randomized to receive placebo or repaglinide (titrated from 0.5 mg bid to a maximum of 4 mg bid). At the end of the 10-week treatment period, mean HbA_{1c} levels had decreased by 2.1% in the repaglinide group, relative to placebo ($p<0.002$). Reductions in fasting (70 mg/dl) and postprandial (112 mg/dl) blood glucose levels were also observed in patients treated with repaglinide, while no significant changes were observed with placebo (Balfour & Faulds, 1998). Similar results were reported for an 18-week, randomized, placebo-controlled, dose-titration study conducted in 99 patients with type 2 diabetes (Goldberg et al., 1998). In this study, doses of repaglinide (0.25 to 8 mg tid with meals) were adjusted to achieve target fasting plasma glucose levels of 90–160 mg/dl. At endpoint, mean HbA_{1c} was reduced by 0.5% in patients receiving repaglinide in comparison to an increase of 1.2% in patients receiving placebo ($p<0.0001$).

Repaglinide has demonstrated efficacy comparable to or greater than the sulfonylureas in achieving glycemic control. In an open-label, randomized, 12-week comparative study conducted in 44 patients previously receiving sulfonylurea therapy, repaglinide (titrated from 0.5 mg to 2 mg bid) significantly reduced postprandial (29 mg/dl) but not fasting blood glucose levels relative to baseline, while glibenclamide (up to 15 mg/day) significantly reduced fasting but not postprandial values (Wolffenbuttel et al., 1993). Mean HbA_{1c} levels did not change significantly in either treatment group. These observations suggest that repaglinide affects glycemic control primarily by its postprandial action. In a 14-week, randomized, double-blind study of repaglinide (up to 4 mg tid) and glibenclamide (up to 10.5 mg/day) in 195 type 2 diabetic patients previously treated with sulfonylurea therapy, significantly lower mean blood glucose and postprandial blood glucose levels were observed in the repaglinide group than in the glibenclamide group at endpoint (Balfour & Faulds, 1998). Mean HbA$_{1c}$ levels decreased by 0.3% and 0.4% from baseline in the repaglinide and glibenclamide groups, respectively; corresponding changes in fasting blood glucose were -52 mg/dl and -61 mg/dl.

In one-year trials, repaglinide therapy resulted in glycemic control equivalent to each of the three sulfonylurea therapies used as comparators. Comparable effects were also observed for repaglinide (0.5 to 4.0 mg tid) and glibenclamide (1.75 to 10.5 mg/day) in a double-blind trial conducted in 424 patients treated for one year (Scrip No. 2371, 1998). At endpoint, similar increases in HbA$_{1c}$ and fasting plasma glucose were observed between the two treatment groups, and the overall safety and incidence of hypoglycemia did not differ significantly in patients treated with repaglinide or glibenclamide.

In another one-year, comparative trial of repaglinide (n=81) and glipizide (n=175), patients were titrated to a target fasting plasma glucose level of 79 to 158 mg/dl (Scrip No. 2371, 1998). Patients receiving repaglinide at doses of 0.5 to 4.0 mg with each meal demonstrated a smaller increase in HbA$_{1c}$ from baseline than patients receiving maximum dose glipizide. This difference did achieve statistical significance ($p<0.05$), but the trial was not designed to show superiority. In addition, glipizide was associated with a higher number of hypoglycemic events than repaglinide (19% versus 15%), although this difference was not statistically significant. Collectively, these studies suggest that with the dose regimens used, repaglinide is at least as effective as the sulfonylureas in the achievement and maintenance of glycemic control.

Results of a multicenter, randomized trial indicated that combination therapy with repaglinide and metformin has synergistic effects on glycemic control (Balfour & Faulds, 1998). In 83 patients inadequately controlled by metformin monotherapy, the addition of repaglinide at doses of 0.5 to 4 mg tid for 3 months provided significantly better glycemic control than either therapy alone. Mean HbA$_{1c}$ was reduced by 1.4% in patients receiving combination therapy, relative to decreases of 0.3% with metformin alone and 0.4% with repaglinide alone. Similarly, greater changes in fasting blood glucose were observed with combination therapy (-39 mg/dl) than with metformin (-5 mg/dl) or repaglinide (-9 mg/dl) monotherapy. Trials of repaglinide in combination with troglitazone therapy are currently underway (Scrip No. 2371, 1998).

The most common adverse event associated with repaglinide therapy is mild to moderate hypoglycemia (Goldberg et al., 1998). While there is some indication that repaglinide may have a lower risk of hypoglycemia than sulfonylurea therapy, further evidence will be necessary to confirm this finding (Wolffenbuttel et al., 1993). One study reported that repaglinide therapy did not result in hypoglycemia if a meal (and the mealtime dose) were skipped, which could enhance patient convenience and safety in comparison to sulfonylurea treatment (Balfour & Faulds, 1998).

In several of the one-year, active control studies, more acute cardiovascular events were observed in the groups treated with repaglinide than in those treated with the sulfonylurea comparator (Fleming, in press). A proposed large, simple trial is expected to resolve this issue in phase IV (The Pink Sheet, January 5, 1998). As repaglinide is metabolized by CYP3A4, potential drug interactions may be observed with other compounds metabolized by this enzymatic pathway. Repaglinide is currently approved for use as both monotherapy and in combination with metformin in patients with type 2 diabetes.

CONCLUSIONS

The therapeutic options available to diabetic patients have expanded considerably within the past decade. Novel drug classes including the biguanides, α-glucosidase inhibitors, thiazolidinediones, and meglitinides have emerged as effective and well-tolerated therapies for improving metabolic control. A possible refinement of sulfonylurea therapy is provided by glimepiride, which may have a more favorable pharmacodynamic profile than previous compounds of this class. Finally, the increased variety of compounds has given rise to new combination therapies, which may result in better glycemic control than can be achieved with monotherapy. Although no strategy to date can be considered optimal, and the attainment and maintenance of euglycemia without significant side effects remains a challenging goal in many patients, the advancements of the past decade have provided a new generation of promising approaches for the treatment of diabetes. Long-term studies that examine major clinical outcomes, such as mortality and diabetic complications, are still needed to define the ultimate value of these approaches.

References

Antonucci T, Whitcomb R, McLain R, Lockwood D, Norris RM. Impaired glucose tolerance is normalized by treatment with the thiazolidinedione troglitazone. *Diabetes Care* 1997; **20**(2): 188–193.

Azen SP, Peters RK, Berkowitz K, Kjos S, Xiang A, Buchanan TA. TRIPOD (Troglitazone In the Prevention Of Diabetes): a randomized, placebo-controlled trial of troglitazone in women with prior gestational diabetes mellitus. *Control Clin Trials* 1998; **19**(2): 217–231.

Bailey CJ, Turner RC. Metformin. *N Engl J Med* 1996; **334**(9): 574–579.

Balfour JA, Faulds D. Repaglinide. *Drugs Aging* 1998; **13**(2): 173–180.

Bloomgarden ZT. Obesity, diabetes prevention, and type 1 diabetes. American Diabetes Association Annual Meeting, 1997. *Diabetes Care* 1997; **20**(12): 1913–1917.

Buse J, Gumbiner B, Mathias NP, Nelson DM, Faja BW, Whitcomb RW. Troglitazone use in insulin-treated type 2 diabetic patients. The Troglitazone Insulin Study Group. *Diabetes Care* 1998b; **21**(9): 1455–1461.

Buse J, Hart K, Minasi L. The PROTECT Study: final results of a large multicenter postmarketing study in patients with type 2 diabetes. Precose Resolution of Optimal Titration to Enhance Current Therapies. *Clin Ther* 1998a; **20**(2): 257–269.

Campbell IW, Menzies DG, Chalmers J, McBain AM, Brown IR. One year comparative trial of metformin and glipizide in type 2 diabetes mellitus. *Diabete Metab* 1994; **20**(4): 394–400.

Chiasson JL, Josse RG, Hunt JA, Palmason C, Rodger NW, Ross SA, Ryan EA, Tan MH, Wolever MS. The efficacy of acarbose in the treatment of patients with non-insulin-dependent diabetes mellitus. *Ann Intern Med* 1994; **121**: 928–935.

Clarke BF, Campbell IW. Comparison of metformin and chlorpropamide in non-obese, maturity-onset diabetics uncontrolled by diet. *BMJ* 1977; **2**(6102): 1576–1578.

Coniff RF, Shapiro JA, Robbins D, Kleinfield R, Seaton TB, Beisswenger P, McGill JB. Reduction of glycosylated hemoglobin and postprandial hyperglycemia by acarbose in patients with NIDDM. A placebo-controlled dose-comparison study. *Diabetes Care* 1995a; **18**(6): 817–824.

Coniff RF, Shapiro JA, Seaton TB, Bray GA. Multicenter, placebo-controlled trial comparing acarbose (BAY g 5421) with placebo, tolbutamide, and tolbutamide-plus-acarbose in non-insulin-dependent diabetes mellitus. *Am J Med* 1995b; **98**: 443–451.

Coniff RF, Shapiro JA, Seaton TB. Long-term efficacy and safety of acarbose in the treatment of obese subjects with non-insulin-dependent diabetes mellitus. *Arch Intern Med* 1994; **154**: 2442–2448.

DeFronzo RA, Goodman AM, Multicenter Metformin Study Group. Efficacy of metformin in patients with non-insulin-dependent diabetes mellitus. *N Engl J Med* 1995; **333**: 541–549.

Dills DG, Schneider J, The Glimepiride/Glibenclamide Research Group. Clinical evaluation of glimepiride versus glibenclamide in NIDDM in a double-blind comparative study. *Horm Metab Res* 1996; **28**: 426–429.

Dimitriadis G, Hatziagelaki K, Ladas S, Linos A, Hillebrand I, Raptis S. Effects of prolonged administration of two new alpha-glucosidase inhibitors on blood glucose control, insulin requirements and breath hydrogen excretion in patients with insulin-dependent diabetes mellitus. *Eur J Clin Invest* 1988; **18**(1): 33–38.

Dimitriadis G, Raptis S, Raptis A, Hatziagelaki E, Mitrakou A, Halvatsiotis P, Ladas S, Hillebrand I. Effects of two new alpha-glucosidase inhibitors on glycemic control in patients with insulin-dependent diabetes mellitus. *Klin Wochenschr* 1986; **64**(9): 405–410.

Dornan TL, Heller SR, Peck GM, Tattersall RB. Double-blind evaluation of efficacy and tolerability of metformin in NIDDM. *Diabetes Care* 1991; **14**(4): 342–344.

Draeger KE, Wernicke-Panten K, Lomp HJ, Roβkamp R. Long-term treatment of type 2 diabetic patients with the new oral antidiabetic agent glimepiride (Amaryl®): a double-blind comparison with glibenclamide. *Horm Metab Res* 1996; **28**: 419–425.

Fleming GA. Current FDA philosophy on approving drugs for diabetic therapy. *Am Heart J*, in press.

Fonseca VA, Valiquett TR, Huang SM, Ghazzi MN, Whitcomb RW. Troglitazone monotherapy improves glycemic control in patients with type 2 diabetes mellitus: a randomized, controlled study. The Troglitazone Study Group. *J Clin Endocrinol Metab* 1998; **83**(9): 3169–3176.

Fuhlendorff J, Rorsman P, Kofod H, Brand CL, Rolin B, MacKay P, Shymko R, Carr RD. Stimulation of insulin release by repaglinide and glibenclamide involves both common and distinct processes. *Diabetes* 1998; **47**(3): 345–351.

Ghazzi MN, Perez JE, Antonucci TK, Driscoll JH, Huang SM, Faja BW, The Troglitazone Study Group, Whitcomb RW. Cardiac and glycemic benefits of troglitazone treatment in NIDDM. *Diabetes* 1997; **46**: 433–439.

Giugliano D, Quatraro A, Consoli G, Minei A, Ceriello A, De Rosa N, D'Onofrio F. Metformin for obese, insulin-treated diabetic patients: improvement in glycaemic control and reduction of metabolic risk factors. *Eur J Clin Pharmacol* 1993; **44**(2): 107–112.

Goldberg RB, Einhorn D, Lucas CP, Rendell MS, Damsbo P, Huang WC, Strange P, Brodows RG. A randomized placebo-controlled trial of repaglinide in the treatment of type 2 diabetes. *Diabetes Care* 1998; **21**(11): 1897–1903.

Goldberg RB, Holvey SM, Schneider J, The Glimepiride Protocol #201 Study Group. A dose-response study of glimepiride in patients with NIDDM who have previously received sulfonylurea therapy. *Diabetes Care* 1996; **19**(8): 849–856.

Hanefield M, Fischer S, Schulze J, Spengler M, Wargenau M, Schollberg K, Fucker K. Therapeutic potentials of acarbose a first-line drug in NIDDM insufficiently treated with diet alone. *Diabetes Care* 1991; **14**(8): 732–737.

Haupt E, Knick B, Koschinsky T, Liebermeister H, Schneider J, Hirche H. Oral antidiabetic combination therapy with sulphonylureas and metformin. *Diabete Metab* 1991; **17**(1 part 2): 224–231.

Henry RR. Thiazolidinediones. *Endocrinol Metab Clin North Am* 1997; **26**(3): 553–573.

Hermann LS, Bitzen PO, Kjellstrom T, Lindgarde F, Schersten B. Comparative efficacy of metformin and glibenclamide in patients with non-insulin-dependent diabetes mellitus. *Diabete Metab* 1991; **17**(1 Part 2): 201–208.

Hermann LS, Schersten B, Bitzen PO, Kjellstrom T, Lindgarde F, Melander A. Therapeutic comparison of metformin and sulfonylurea, alone and in various combinations. A double-blind controlled study. *Diabetes Care* 1994; **17**(10): 1100–1109.

Horton ES, Whitehouse F, Ghazzi MN, Veneable TC, Whitcomb RW. Troglitazone in combination with sulfonylurea restores glycemic control in patients with type 2 diabetes. The Troglitazone Study Group. *Diabetes Care* 1998; **21**(9): 1462–1469.

Inzucchi SE, Maggs DG, Spollet GR, Page SL, Rife FS, Walton V, Shulman GI. Efficacy and metabolic effects of metformin and troglitazone in type II diabetes mellitus. *N Engl J Med* 1998; **338**(13): 867–872.

Iwamoto Y, Kosaka K, Kuzuya T, Akanuma Y, Shigeta Y, Kaneko T. Effects of troglitazone: a new hypoglycemic agent in patients with NIDDM poorly controlled by diet therapy. *Diabetes Care* 1996a; **19**(2): 151–156.

Iwamoto Y, Kosaka K, Kuzuya T, Akanuma Y, Shigeta Y, Kaneko T. Effect of combination therapy of troglitazone and sulphonylureas in patients with type 2 diabetes who were poorly controlled by sulphonylurea therapy alone. *Diabet Med* 1996b; **13**(4): 365–370.

Johnson MD, Campbell LK, Campbell RK. Troglitazone: review and assessments of its role in the treatment of patients with impaired glucose tolerance and diabetes mellitus. *Ann Pharmacother* 1998; **32**: 337–348.

Johnston PS, Coniff RF, Hoogwerf BJ, Santiago JV, Pi-Sunyer FX, Krol A. Effects of the carbohydrase inhibitor miglitol in sulfonylurea-treated patients. *Diabetes Care* 1994; **17**(1): 20–29.

Johnston PS, Lebovitz HE, Coniff RF, Simonson DC, Raskin P, Munera CL. Advantages of alpha-glucosidase inhibition as monotherapy in elderly type 2 diabetic patients. *J Clin Endocrinol Metab* 1998; **83**(5): 1515–1522.

Kelley DE, Bidot P, Freedman Z, Haag B, Podlecki D, Rendell M, Schimel D, Weiss S, Taylor T, Krol A, et al. Efficacy and safety of acarbose in insulin-treated patients with type 2 diabetes. *Diabetes Care* 1998; **21**: 2056–2061.

Kumar S, Boulton AJ, Beck-Nielsen H, Berthezene F, Muggeo M, Persson B, Spinas GA, Donoghue S, Lettis S, Stewart-Long P. Troglitazone, an insulin action enhancer, improves metabolic control in NIDDM patients. Troglitazone Study Group. *Diabetologia* 1996; **39**(6): 701–709.

Kumar S, Prange A, Schulze J, Lettis S, Barnett AH. Troglitazone, an insulin action enhancer, improves glycaemic control and insulin sensitivity in elderly type 2 diabetic patients. *Diabet Med* 1998; **15**(9): 772–779.

Maggs DG, Buchanan TA, Burant CF, Cline G, Gumbiner B, Hsueh WA, Inzucchi S, Kelley D, Nolan J, Olefsky JM, et al. Metabolic effects of troglitazone monotherapy in type 2 diabetes mellitus. A randomized, double-blind, placebo-controlled trial. *Ann Intern Med* 1998; **128**(3): 176–185.

Misbin RI, Green L, Stadel BV, Gueriguian JL, Gubbi A, Fleming GA. Lactic acidosis in patients with diabetes treated with metformin. *N Engl J Med* 1998; **338**(4): 265–266.

Mitrakou A, Tountas N, Raptis AE, Bauer RJ, Schulz H, Raptis SA. Long-term effectiveness of a new α-glucosidase inhibitor (BAY m1099-miglitol) in insulin-treated type 2 diabetes mellitus. *Diabet Med* 1998; **15**: 657–660.

Müller G, Hartz D, Pünter J, Ökonomopulos R, Kramer W. Differential interaction of glimepiride and glibenclamide with the β-cell sulfonylurea receptor. I. Binding characteristics. *Biochem Biophys Acta* 1994; **1191**: 267–277.

Nagi DK, Yudkin JS. Effects of metformin on insulin resistance, risk factors for cardiovascular disease, and plasminogen activator inhibitor in NIDDM subjects. A study of two ethnic groups. *Diabetes Care* 1993; **16**(4): 621–629.

Nolan JJ, Ludvik B, Beerdsen P, Joyce M, Olefsky J. Improvement in glucose tolerance and insulin resistance in obese subjects treated with troglitazone. *N Engl J Med* 1994; **331**(18): 1188–1193.

Pagano G, Marena S, Corgiat-Mansin L, Cravero F, Giorda C, Bozza M, Rossi CM. Comparison of miglitol and glibenclamide in diet-treated type 2 diabetic patients. *Diabete Metab* 1995; **21**: 162–167.

Physician's Desk Reference, 53rd ed. *Precose.*® Montvale, NJ: Medical Economics Company, 1999, pp. 667–669.

The Pink Sheet. Bristol *Glucophage* adds congestive heart failure contraindication; public citizen reviewing BMS *phase IV* protocol, sues FDA for *Redux* post-marketing protocol. January 26, 1998, p. 11.

The Pink Sheet. Novo Nordisk *Prandin* launch to follow announcement of co-promotion partner in Spring; antidiabetic approved for monotherapy and with metformin. January 5; 1998, p. 15.

The Pink Sheet. Warner-Lambert *Rezulin* liver toxicity risk estimate is 1 in 60,000. August 3, 1998, p. 20.

Riddle MC, Schneider J, Glimepiride Combination Group. Beginning insulin treatment of obese patients with evening 70/30 insulin plus glimepiride versus insulin alone. *Diabetes Care* 1998; 21(7): 1052–1057.

Robinson AC, Burke J, Robinson S, Johnston DG, Elkeles RS. The effects of metformin on glycemic control and serum lipids in insulin-treated NIDDM patients with suboptimal metabolic control. *Diabetes Care* 1998; 21(5): 701–705.

Rosenstock J, Brown A, Fischer F, Jain A, Littlejohn T, Nadeau D, Sussman A, Taylor T, Krol A, Magner J. Efficacy and safety of acarbose in metformin-treated patients with type 2 diabetes. *Diabetes Care* 1998; 21: 2050–2055.

Schade DS, Jovanovic L, Schneider J. A placebo-controlled, randomized study of glimepiride in patients with type 2 diabetes mellitus for whom diet therapy is unsuccessful. *J Clin Pharmacol* 1998; 38(7): 636–641.

Schneider J, Chaikin P. Glimepiride safety: results of placebo-controlled, dose regimen, and active-controlled trials. *Postgrad Med* 1997; Jun, Special Report: 33–44.

Schwartz S, Raskin P, Fonseca V, Graveline JF. Effect of troglitazone in insulin-treated patients with type II diabetes mellitus. Troglitazone and Exogenous Insulin Study Group. *N Engl J Med* 1998; 338(13): 861–866.

Scrip No. 2357. Call to ban troglitazone in US. July 31, 1998; p. 22.

Scrip No. 2371. Repaglinide offers new approach to diabetes therapy. September 18, 1998; p 22.

Scrip No. 2390. Troglitazone for diabetes prevention. November 25, 1998; p. 19.

Segal P, Feig PU, Schernthaner G, Ratzmann KP, Rybka J, Petzinna D, Berlin C. The efficacy and safety of miglitol therapy compared with glibenclamide in patients with NIDDM inadequately controlled by diet alone. *Diabetes Care* 1997; 20(5): 687–691.

Sonnenberg GE, Garg DC, Weidler DJ, Dixon RM, Jaber LA, Bowen AJ, DeChemey GS, Mullican WS, Stonesifer LD. Short-term comparison of once- versus twice-daily administration of glimepiride in patients with non-insulin-dependent diabetes mellitus. *Ann Pharmacother* 1997; 31(6): 671–676.

Sparano N, Seaton TL. Troglitazone in type II diabetes mellitus. *Pharmacotherapy* 1998; **18**(3): 539–548.

UKPDS Group. United Kingdom Prospective Diabetes Study 24: a 6-year, randomized, controlled trial comparing sulfonylurea, insulin, and metformin therapy in patients with newly diagnosed type 2 diabetes that could not be controlled with diet therapy. *Ann Intern Med* 1998a; **128**(3): 165–175.

UKPDS Group. Effect of intensive blood-glucose control with metformin on complications in overweight patients with type 2 diabetes (UKPDS 34). *Lancet* 1998b; **352**(9131): 854–865.

UKPDS Group. Intensive blood-glucose control with sulphonylureas or insulin compared with conventional treatment and risk of complications in patients with type 2 diabetes (UKPDS 33). *Lancet* 1998c; **352**: 837–853.

University Group Diabetes Program. A study of the effects of hypoglycemic agents on vascular complications in patients with adult-onset diabetes. V. Evaluation of phenformin therapy. *Diabetes* 1975; **24**(Suppl 1): 65–184.

Wolffenbuttel BH, Nijst L, Sels JP, Menheere PP, Muller PG, Kruseman AC. Effects of a new oral hypoglycemic agent, repaglinide, on metabolic control in sulphonylurea-treated patients with NIDDM. *Eur J Clin Pharmacol* 1993; **45**(2): 113–116.

Yee HS, Fong NT. A review of the safety and efficacy of acarbose in diabetes mellitus. *Pharmacotherapy* 1996; **16**(5): 792–805.

8

REVIEW OF ANTIDIABETIC COMPOUNDS IN THE PIPELINE

The pipeline for antidiabetic compounds illustrates the growing diversity of treatment strategies for this disease. Although some of these compounds are new members of existing drug classes (e.g., α-glucosidase inhibitors, thiazolidinediones), others are designed to have novel underlying mechanisms of action. Moreover, the first drugs designed to directly prevent or treat diabetic complications have opened the door to a wholly new approach to treatment, and could fundamentally change the therapeutic options for patients with this disease (Table 8.1).

NOVEL ANTIDIABETIC COMPOUNDS: IMPROVEMENT OF GLYCEMIC CONTROL

Voglibose

Voglibose is a novel α-glucosidase inhibitor under investigation as a treatment for type 2 diabetic patients inadequately controlled by diet therapy alone. Like other members of its class, voglibose delays the digestion of disaccharides and complex carbohydrates in the intestines through the inhibition of α-glucosidase enzymes, thus reducing postprandial glucose excursions. However, voglibose can be distinguished from acarbose in that it is substantially more potent against disaccharidase, and less potent against pancreatic α-amylase (Matsuo et al., 1992). Studies in diabetic animals have indicated that voglibose may also reduce visceral fat deposits and free fatty acid levels, which could be particularly beneficial for obese diabetic patients (Kobatake et al., 1989). Doses of 0.2 to 0.3 mg tid are currently approved in Japan for patients with type 2 diabetes.

An open-label, prospective study of voglibose was conducted in 27 type 2 diabetic patients who were hospitalized due to inadequate glycemic control with diet and/or sulfonylurea therapy (Matsumoto et al., 1998). Fourteen of the patients received additional therapy with voglibose 0.2 mg tid before meals, while the remaining patients continued with their previous antidiabetic regimen and served as a control group. Doses of voglibose and the dietary regimen were unchanged throughout the study, while doses of sulfonylurea therapy (glibenclamide or gliclazide) were adjusted to achieve target levels of fasting (<140 mg/dl) and postprandial (<200 mg/dl) plasma glucose. After four weeks, patients receiving voglibose demonstrated significantly lower daily glycemic excursions than control patients

Table 8.1 - The pipeline for antidiabetic compounds

Compound	Therapeutic Class	Indication
voglibose	α-glucosidase inhibitor	type 2 diabetes
pramlintide	amylin analog	type 1, type 2 diabetes
GLP-1	gut hormone	type 2 diabetes
rosiglitazone	thiazolidinedione	type 2 diabetes
pioglitazone	thiazolidinedione	type 2 diabetes
pimagedine	anti-glycation compound	diabetic nephropathy
zenarestat	aldose reductase inhibitor	diabetic neuropathy
zopolrestat	aldose reductase inhibitor	diabetic neuropathy
bimoclomol	anti-ischemic compound	diabetic complications
acetyl-L-carnitine	carnitine activator	diabetic neuropathy
EXO-226	anti-glycation compound	diabetic nephropathy

receiving diet and/or sulfonylureas alone ($p<0.05$). These results were largely due to an attenuation of postprandial hyperglycemia in voglibose-treated patients.

In another open-label study, a total of 36 type 2 diabetic patients on sulfonylurea or insulin therapy who demonstrated inadequate glycemic control or symptoms of hypoglycemia received adjunct therapy with voglibose (0.2 mg tid before each meal) for up to 12 weeks (Okada et al., 1996a). Patients who had exhibited regular symptoms of hypoglycemia on their previous therapeutic regimen also received a dose reduction. The addition of voglibose, accompanied by decreased dosages of sulfonylurea or insulin therapy, resulted in the elimination of hypoglycemia without a loss of overall glycemic control. Combination therapy with voglibose and unchanged doses of sulfonylureas or insulin did not result in significant changes in postprandial blood glucose or HbA_{1c} levels. Thus, the addition of voglibose may allow patients to reduce sulfonylurea or insulin doses, and potentially the incidence of hypoglycemia, without compromising overall metabolic control. An open, prospective study also found that in ten patients receiving voglibose (0.1 mg tid with meals) for 4 weeks, the addition of low-dose tolbutamide for another 4 weeks resulted in significant reductions in HbA_{1c} in comparison to voglibose alone. No side effects, including hypoglycemia or hyperinsulinemia, were reported during the course of the study (Okada et al., 1996b).

Voglibose has also been shown to reduce insulin resistance and dyslipidemia in hyperinsulinemic non-diabetic individuals. In one study, 16 subjects with hyperinsulinemia, 8 of whom also had impaired glucose tolerance, received treatment with 0.2 mg tid voglibose prior to each meal for 12 weeks. Voglibose therapy resulted in significant improvements in postprandial plasma glucose and insulin, as well as overall triglyceride levels (Shinozaki et al., 1996). In addition, a steady state plasma glucose test, performed in 8 of these subjects (4 with impaired glucose tolerance) prior to and at the end of the voglibose treatment period, demonstrated an improvement in insulin sensitivity and glucose utilization. These results suggest that voglibose may have indirect beneficial effects on insulin sensitivity in addition to its direct activity on the gastrointestinal system. However, an open-label, prospective study conducted in 27 type 2 diabetic patients receiving diet or sulfonylurea therapy found that the addition of 0.2 mg tid voglibose reduced daily glycemic excursions but did not appear to have an effect of insulin sensitivity in this population (Matsumoto et al., 1998).

Like other members of its class, voglibose is associated with mild to moderate gastrointestinal adverse events, such as diarrhea, flatulence, and abdominal distension (Shinozaki et al., 1996; Goke et al., 1995). These effects appear to decline over the course of treatment, and have not generally been associated with early discontinuation from therapy in published trials. Although reports of liver function abnormalities have emerged from adverse event monitoring of voglibose in Japan (Scrip No. 2322, 1998), these events occurred in a small number of patients. This compound is currently in phase III clinical trials.

Pramlintide

Amylin, an amino acid peptide hormone co-secreted with insulin from pancreatic β-cells, is involved in the reduction of postprandial glucose levels through the suppression of glucagon secretion and the modulation of gastric emptying (Scherbaum, 1998). As levels of this hormone have been shown to be reduced or absent in patients with type 1 or late stage type 2 diabetes, replacement therapy has emerged as a potential option to improve glycemic control (Enoki et al., 1992; Koda et al., 1992). However, human amylin has a tendency to aggregate into insoluble fibrils *ex vivo*, making it a poor candidate for development as a therapeutic agent. To address this problem, the amylin analog pramlintide was developed, which retains the biological activity of the human hormone without its propensity to aggregate in solution.

The subcutaneous or intravenous administration of pramlintide prior to meals has been shown to effectively delay the gastric emptying of both solids and liquids in patients with type 1 diabetes (Kong et al., 1998; Kong et al., 1997). Subcutaneous injections of 30, 100, or 300 µg pramlintide, administered 30 minutes before meals for 14 days, also significantly reduced postprandial hyperglycemia in type 1 diabetic patients (Kolterman et al., 1996). In addition, the intravenous infusion of pramlintide (50 µg/h for 5 h) was reported to reduce postprandial glucose concentrations following a standardized meal but not following an intravenous glucose load, consistent with its local effects on the gastrointestinal tract (Kolterman et al., 1995).

The reduction of postprandial glucose levels observed with pramlintide also appears to improve overall glycemic control in diabetic patients. In a randomized, double-blind, placebo-controlled study, 168 patients with type 1 diabetes received subcutaneous pramlintide at doses of 10, 30, or 100 µg qid or placebo in addition to their regular insulin regimen for 14 days (Thompson et al., 1997a). Improvements in postprandial glucose responses were observed at the 1 and 2 week timepoints for patients receiving 30 or 100 µg qid pramlintide, while the 30 µg qid dose was also associated with a reduction in 24-h mean glucose concentrations (34 mg/dl) compared with placebo (0.5 mg/dl) at endpoint. Similar results were observed in another double-blind, placebo-controlled trial (Thompson et al.,

1997b) in which 215 type 1 diabetic patients were randomized to receive placebo or one of four dose regimens of subcutaneous pramlintide for four weeks: 30 µg qid (with breakfast, lunch, dinner, and an evening snack); 30 µg tid (with breakfast, lunch, and dinner); 30 µg tid (with breakfast, dinner, and an evening snack); or 60 µg bid (with breakfast and dinner). At endpoint, treatment with 30 µg qid pramlintide resulted in a significant improvement in mean 24-h plasma glucose levels (-25 mg/dl) in comparison to placebo (increase of 5 mg/dl; $p<0.009$ pramlintide versus placebo). In addition, reductions in serum fructosamine were observed in patients receiving all four dose regimens of pramlintide, although only the mean improvement in the 30 µg qid group was significantly greater than placebo ($p<0.003$). Several patients receiving pramlintide were able to reduce their dosages of short-acting insulin during the study, while patients receiving placebo reported a mean increase.

Pramlintide has also been shown to improve metabolic control in patients with type 2 diabetes receiving insulin therapy. For example, Thompson et al. (1998) conducted a 4-week, randomized, double-blind, placebo-controlled study comparing 30 µg qid, 60 µg tid, and 60 µg qid pramlintide with placebo in 203 insulin-treated type 2 diabetic patients. In this study, significant improvements in serum fructosamine were observed with all three doses of pramlintide in comparison to placebo at endpoint. Moreover, significant reductions in HbA$_{1c}$ relative to baseline were observed for patients receiving pramlintide 30 µg qid (0.53%), 60 µg tid (0.58%), and 60 µg qid (0.51%) in comparison to patients receiving placebo (0.27%). Reductions in body weight and mean fasting total cholesterol were also reported for the 60 µg tid and 60 µg qid pramlintide treatment groups.

Initial results from two 6-month, phase III trials indicated that 90 µg tid pramlintide as an adjunct to insulin therapy failed to achieve significant reductions in fasting plasma glucose levels (Scrip No. 2382, 1998). However, significant reductions in blood glucose and HbA$_{1c}$ were observed with lower, well-tolerated doses of pramlintide, suggesting that dosage and regimen may have affected these results. Moreover, open-label extension studies showed that those type 1 patients who were "responders" (HbA$_{1c}$ reductions of at least 0.5% after 4 weeks of therapy) demonstrated greater average HbA$_{1c}$ reductions at 6 months (0.9%), 12 months (0.8%) and 18 months (0.8%; Scrip No. 2407, 1999). In type 2 diabetic patients, average reductions in HbA$_{1c}$ in patients who demonstrated glucose-lowering effects at 6 months were 0.7–0.8% at 6 months, 0.7% at 12 months, and 0.4–0.6% at 24 months, while corresponding reductions in responders were 1.1–1.2%, 0.9–1.0%, and 0.9%, respectively.

Consistent with its mechanism of action, the most common adverse events associated with pramlintide therapy are gastrointestinal effects including nausea, anorexia, and dyspepsia (Thompson et al., 1997a, 1997b). These events appear to improve following the first week of therapy. The incidence of hypoglycemia has been reported to be similar in patients receiving pramlintide or placebo in most studies. One intriguing aspect of amylin therapy is that its action on gastric emptying is reversed by insulin-induced hypoglycemia, suggesting a protective mechanism against this adverse event (Gedulin & Young, 1998).

GLP-1

The truncated form of the gut hormone, GLP-1 (GLP-1 [7–36/7]), has demonstrated multiple anti-hyperglycemic effects in diabetic patients, including the enhancement of insulin secretion in response to glucose, slowing of gastric emptying, and suppression of glucagon production (Drucker, 1998). These effects suggest that GLP-1 may be effective in improving metabolic control in patients with type 2 diabetes without inducing hypoglycemia, a potential advantage over currently available antidiabetic therapies (Byrne and Goke, 1996).

As GLP-1 is released into the bloodstream following meals, it is thought to be involved in the suppression of postprandial hyperglycemia. Several small clinical studies have reported that GLP-1 significantly reduced or even prevented postprandial glucose excursions in type 2 diabetic patients following subcutaneous or intravenous administration (Todd et al., 1998; Todd et al., 1997; Dupre et al., 1995; Nathan et al., 1992). In addition, the intravenous administration of GLP-1 was shown to normalize fasting plasma glucose levels in overtly hyperglycemic type 2 diabetic patients inadequately controlled by diet, sulfonylurea, or metformin therapy (Nauck et al., 1998a). Even in advanced type 2 diabetic patients with secondary sulfonylurea failure who had previously been treated with insulin for several years, the intravenous administration of GLP-1 significantly reduced fasting plasma glucose in comparison to placebo (Nauck et al., 1998b).

However, the intravenous administration of GLP-1 is impossible for routine therapy, and subcutaneous injection may limit patient convenience and compliance. To address this issue, a buccal tablet form of GLP-1 has been developed. In an initial study, eight healthy subjects demonstrated potentially therapeutic plasma levels of GLP-1 following the administration of a single mucoadhesive buccal GLP-1 tablet (Gutniak et al., 1996). Another study conducted in ten type 2 diabetic patients found that treatment with buccal GLP-1 tablets resulted in marked insulinotropic and glucose-lowering effects during the 2-hour period following administration, both in the fasting state and after a mixed meal (Gutniak et al., 1997). Thus, buccal tablets may be a feasible and more convenient alternative to parenteral GLP-1 therapy. In addition, as GLP-1 undergoes rapid enzymatic degradation *in vivo*, resulting in low overall bioavailability, analogs with prolonged metabolic stability are also under investigation at this time (Deacon et al., 1998; Ritzel et al., 1995).

GLP-1 is not associated with adverse events at doses producing near-physiological levels of the hormone. At higher doses, however, dizziness, chills, nausea, and vomiting have been observed in healthy subjects (Ritzel et al., 1995). Nausea, vomiting, and dizziness have also been reported in studies of GLP-1 in the patient population (Nauck et al., 1996). In addition, a near-complete inhibition of gastric emptying was observed in diabetic patients who received intravenous GLP-1 following a liquid meal (Willms et al., 1996). While a slowing of gastric emptying may help to reduce postprandial glucose excursions, such extreme effects are clearly not desirable, and may be preventable with proper dosing or with new formulations.

Rosiglitazone

Rosiglitazone is a novel member of the thiazolidinedione class currently under investigation for the treatment of type 2 diabetes. Like troglitazone, rosiglitazone binds to the peroxisome proliferator-activated receptor-γ, which is involved in the regulation of glucose and fatty acid metabolism (Young et al., 1998). Rosiglitazone has demonstrated the capacity to improve insulin sensitivity and glucose tolerance in high-fat fed rats (Oakes et al., 1994) and genetically diabetic mice (Connor et al., 1997). These effects are potentially due to the reduction of serum free fatty acid levels, which can contribute to insulin resistance in peripheral tissues (Souza et al., 1998; Oakes et al., 1997; Oakes et al., 1994). Moreover, rosiglitazone treatment was reported to delay or prevent the development of nephropathy and pancreatic cell abnormalities in Zucker fatty rats, in addition to slowing the progression of existing complications (Buckingham et al., 1998).

Although few clinical studies have been published at this time, preliminary results of a 26-week, randomized, placebo-controlled phase III trial conducted in 493 type 2 diabetic patients indicated that rosiglitazone significantly improved fasting blood glucose levels at doses of 4 mg/day (-58 mg/dL) and 8 mg/day (-76 mg/dl) relative to placebo (Clinical Investigator News, 1998; Scrip No. 2345, 1998). In addition, HbA_{1c} levels were significantly reduced by 1.2% and 1.5% of total hemoglobin in the 4 mg/day and 8 mg/day groups, respectively.

Overall, side effects appear to be similar between patients receiving rosiglitazone and those receiving placebo (Scrip No. 2345, 1998). Although reports of liver toxicity with troglitazone have raised concerns regarding other thiazolidinedione compounds, no drug reactions leading to jaundice or liver failure have been reported in 1400 patients treated with rosiglitazone for more than one year (Scrip No. 2345, 1998). However, minor anemia, fluid retention, and weight gain were observed in some patients. Two additional pivotal phase III trials assessing the efficacy and safety of rosiglitazone in combination with insulin or metformin are currently underway.

Pioglitazone

Another thiazolidinedione, pioglitazone, is also under investigation as a potentially safer alternative to troglitazone therapy. Pioglitazone has been reported to effectively reverse insulin resistance induced by tumor necrosis factor-α in hepatic cells (Solomon et al., 1997), and to stimulate the expression of glucose transporter mRNA and protein in muscle cells *in vitro* (el-Kebbi et al., 1994). In addition, pioglitazone has been shown to reduce insulin resistance caused by the administration of growth hormone in obese (ob/ob) mice (Towns et al., 1994).

Several clinical trials of pioglitazone in type 2 diabetes are currently underway in Japan. In one study, 20 type 2 diabetic patients treated with diet or sulfonylurea therapy received 30 mg/day pioglitazone for approximately 87 days (Yamasaki et al., 1997). Pioglitazone treatment significantly improved the rate of insulin-stimulated glucose disposal, as measured by a glucose clamp. Moreover, fasting plasma glucose levels and HbA_{1c} were significantly reduced by 38 mg/dl and 0.9%, respectively, over the course of the study. These results suggest that pioglitazone improves overall glycemic control through its beneficial effects on insulin resistance. Additional support for these results was provided by a double-blind, placebo-controlled trial of 30 patients with type 2 diabetes treated with diet alone or sulfonylureas (Kawamori et al., 1998). Patients received either 30 mg/day pioglitazone (n=21) or placebo (n=9) a total of 12 weeks. At the end of the treatment period, a euglycemic, hyperinsulinemic glucose clamp procedure combined with an oral glucose load revealed that pioglitazone significantly reduced insulin resistance by increasing both splanchnic and peripheral glucose uptake, while no effects were observed with placebo.

Early reports indicate that effects on liver enzymes have not been observed in clinical trials of pioglitazone (Scrip No. 2338/39, 1998); however, the full results of these trials will be necessary to evaluate the risk of this potential adverse event.

NOVEL ANTIDIABETIC COMPOUNDS: TREATMENT OR PREVENTION OF DIABETIC COMPLICATIONS

Pimagedine

Pimagedine (aminoguanidine) has been shown to inhibit the formation of advanced glycation end products (AGEs), which are implicated in the development of micro- and macrovascular complications in diabetes. Although the protective effects of pimagedine appear to be predominantly mediated by a reduction in AGE formation (Soulis et al., 1997), this compound also functions as an inhibitor of nitric oxide synthase and oxidative stress, which are potential contributing factors to the development of tissue damage in diabetic patients (Yang et al., 1998). In animal models of diabetes and diabetic complications, treatment with pimagedine resulted in the prevention or reduction of retinopathy (Hammes et al., 1995; Hammes et al., 1994; Hammes et al., 1991) and the amelioration of albuminuria (Edelstein & Brownlee, 1992). Pimagedine also prolonged the survival of diabetic rats made azotemic by renal ablation, suggesting that it has protective effects even in cases of existing renal damage (Friedman et al., 1997). Moreover, pimagedine has demonstrated potential benefits against macroangiopathy, including anti-atherogenic effects in cholesterol-fed rabbits (Panagiotopoulos et al., 1998) and reduced infarct volume in a rat model of focal cerebral ischemia (Zimmerman et al., 1995).

In a double-blind, placebo-controlled, 28-day trial, circulating hemoglobin AGE levels were reduced significantly (by approximately 28%) in patients receiving an average dose of 1200 mg/day pimagedine (n=18) in contrast to no significant change in those receiving placebo (n=8; Makita et al., 1992). To assess the efficacy of pimagedine in diabetic patients with microvascular complications, three pivotal clinical trials have been initiated in North America. ACTION I (A Clinical Trial In Overt Nephropathy) was conducted in 690 patients with type 1 diabetes. Continued data analyses of this trial increasingly support preliminary findings that showed pimagedine therapy provided a statistically significant reduction in urinary protein, LDL cholesterol, and triglycerides, as well as lowered diastolic blood pressure. In addition, the data indicated favorable outcomes in measures of renal function, including creatinine clearance and filtration rate, as well as in the inhibition of the progression of retinopathy. ACTION II was conducted in 599 patients with type 2 diabetes. However, an external monitoring committee recommended the discontinuation of this trial because of an insufficient risk/benefit ratio based upon data currently available at that time (Scrip No. 2320, 1998). A third multicenter trial of patients with early diabetic nephropathy was undertaken in Europe, but was canceled due to slow enrollment and difficulty maintaining a placebo group. Finally, enrollment is also in progress for a trial of pimagedine in type 1 and type 2 diabetic patients with end stage renal disease.

Zenarestat

Zenarestat is an aldose reductase inhibitor which effectively reduces the accumulation of sorbitol and fructose in the nerve, lens, retina, and renal cortex of diabetic rats (Ao et al.,

1991a). These effects have been shown to be correlated with the normalization of myo-inositol levels and the prevention or reduction of various microvascular complications *in vivo*. For example, the intraocular administration of zenarestat resulted in a dose-dependent reduction of cataract formation in diabetic rats, as compared to placebo (Ao et al., 1991b). Moreover, treatment with zenarestat for 17 weeks resulted in the recovery of motor NCV in diabetic rats (Ao et al., 1991a).

Zenarestat was well tolerated in healthy volunteers at single oral doses of 600 mg or twice-daily doses of 300 mg (Kanamaru et al., 1993). In addition, the inhibition of aldose reductase was proportional to plasma concentrations of zenarestat over a dose range of 150 to 600 mg/day. The results of Phase II trials indicated that zenarestat significantly improved NCV and nerve fiber density in diabetic patients (Clinical Investigator News, 1998). Although a previous aldose reductase inhibitor, tolrestat, was withdrawn from the market due to liver toxicity, zenarestat has been well tolerated in diabetic patients, without adverse hepatic effects (Clinical Investigator News, 1998). Phase III trials in patients with diabetic neuropathy are currently underway in the U.S.

Zopolrestat

The aldose reductase inhibitor, zopolrestat, has demonstrated highly potent inhibition of sorbitol *in vitro* and *in vivo* (Mylari et al., 1991). Zopolrestat also protected the rate of myo-inositol influx in rat lenses incubated in a high galactose medium (Beyer-Mears et al., 1997). In diabetic rats receiving zopolrestat for four months, proteinuria was significantly reduced in comparison to age-matched controls, indicating potential beneficial effects on diabetic nephropathy (Beyer-Mears et al., 1996). In addition, zopolrestat had beneficial effects on lens transparency and myo-inositol content, despite an increase in lens glucose, suggesting that it may also be effective in preventing retinopathy. Finally, zopolrestat may help to prevent macrovascular complications, as it reduced sorbitol levels in diabetic rat hearts and resulted in significant protection during ischemia and reperfusion (Ramasamy et al., 1997).

Zopolrestat is currently under clinical investigation for the treatment of diabetic neuropathy. In phase II clinical trials of diabetic patients, zopolrestat significantly improved NCV relative to placebo in a variety of nerve types, with mean gains of approximately 1.0 m/s (The Pink Sheet, November 3, 1997). In addition, interim results of an initial phase III pivotal trial indicated that zopolrestat had a favorable safety and efficacy profile in this study (Scrip No. 2387, 1998).

Acetyl-L-Carnitine

Diabetes is associated with a reduction in plasma levels of L-carnitine, which may contribute to the aberrant metabolism of long-chain fatty acids and their subsequent accumulation in nerve tissues (Ido et al., 1994; De Palo et al., 1981). The extent of L-carnitine depletion has been shown to correlate with reductions in motor NCV in diabetic animals (Arduini et al., 1996). Thus, therapy with the carnitine activator acetyl-L-carnitine (ALC) represents a potential approach to the prevention or treatment of diabetic neuropathy. The oral administration of ALC has been shown to dose-dependently increase serum concentrations of L-carnitine in diabetic rats (Marzo et al., 1993). ALC treatment is also reported to normalize or attenuate the deterioration of NCV in already-impaired diabetic rats, suggesting that it may be useful in treating existing peripheral neuropathic symptoms (Soneru et al., 1997; Cotter et al., 1995; Morabito et al., 1993). Furthermore, ALC prevented alterations in gut peptides such as substance P and vasoactive intestinal polypeptide in diabetic animals, which indicates potential therapeutic benefits against autonomic neuropathy (Gorio et al., 1992).

Few clinical studies of ALC therapy have been published at this time. In an initial single-blind, randomized, placebo-controlled, crossover study, 20 diabetic patients with symptomatic peripheral diabetic neuropathy received intramuscular ALC and placebo for 15 days each, separated by a 2-week washout period (Quatraro et al., 1995). A significantly greater improvement in symptom severity, as measured by a visual analog scale, was reported for ALC in comparison to placebo ($p<0.01$). Similar results were found in a trial of the ALC compound ST200 in 94 patients with painful peripheral neuropathy (Onofrj et al., 1995). In this study, significant improvements in total motility, severity of symptoms on a visual analogue scale, and ratings of objective and subjective efficacy were reported for ST200 in comparison to placebo. The compound was well tolerated over the course of the study. However, preliminary results from a larger, multicenter trial did not support the superiority of ALC over placebo in patients with diabetic neuropathy (Fedele & Giugliano, 1997). Thus, further controlled trials will be necessary to determine the efficacy of this approach.

Bimoclomol

The hydroxylamine derivative, bimoclomol, is a novel cytoprotective agent that has been shown to induce the expression of heat shock proteins *in vivo*. These proteins are thought to maintain cell integrity under pathophysiological conditions, and thus may prevent the development of complications in patients with diabetes. Bimoclomol has demonstrated cytoprotective effects in several animal models of tissue damage, including ischemia in the mouse and wound healing in the diabetic rat (Vigh et al., 1997). The treatment of diabetic rats with bimoclomol also prevented and corrected abnormalities on electroretinograms and visual evoked potentials, which are early indications of retinopathy (Biro et al., 1998). In another study of diabetic rats, the 3-month administration of bimoclomol significantly reduced initial physiological correlates of peripheral neuropathy, including the slowing of nerve conduction and elevated ischemic resistance (Biro et al., 1997). Collectively, these studies suggest that bimoclomol may be an effective therapy for the prevention or treatment of various complications in diabetic patients. This compound is currently in Phase II clinical trials.

EXO-226

EXO-226 is an anti-glycation compound currently under development for the prevention of diabetic nephropathy. Diabetic mice treated with EXO-226 for three months demonstrated a significant reduction in serum glycated protein levels relative to untreated animals, which was associated with a decrease in urine albumin excretion (Clinical Investigator News, July, 1998). EXO-226 also reduced the amount of kidney scarring in this animal model. Moreover, positive results from early phase II clinical trials have been reported which indicate that EXO-226 reduces the blood concentration of glycated protein in diabetic patients, despite abnormally high levels of blood glucose (Scrip No. 2351, 1998).

CONCLUSIONS

Therapeutic development for the treatment of diabetes and its complications has exploded in recent years. Some promising therapies such as protein kinase C inhibitors, glucagon receptor antagonists, synthetic exendin-4, and novel insulin sensitizing compounds and insulin secretagogues are not covered here because little if any clinical data are publicly available. Leptin, related compounds, and other anti-obesity therapies may also provide antidiabetic benefits, but their discussion is deferred.

The pipeline for antidiabetic compounds includes both new members of existing drug classes and novel approaches to therapy. As troubling side effects have emerged for some currently available therapies, many of these compounds have focused on increasing safety and tolerability. Over half of the compounds reviewed in this chapter are designed to prevent or treat the complications of diabetes, reflecting the increasing progress in this area. It is hoped that the development of safer and more effective therapies to improve glycemic control, in combination with compounds for the prevention or treatment of diabetic complications, will result in a significant reduction of morbidity and mortality in patients with diabetes.

References

Ao S, Kikuchi C, Ono T, Notsu Y. Effect of instillation of aldose reductase inhibitor FR74366 on diabetic cataract. *Invest Opthalmol Vis Sci* 1991b; **32**(12): 3078–3083.

Ao S, Shingu Y, Kikuchi C, Takano Y, Nomura K, Fujiwara T, Ohkubo Y, Notsu Y, Yamaguchi I. Characterization of novel aldose reductase inhibitor, FR74366, and its effects on diabetic cataract and neuropathy in the rat. *Metabolism* 1991a; **40**(1): 77–87.

Arduini A, Chiodi P, Bellucci A, Calvani M. Abnormality of nerve conduction in diabetic neuropathy: is there a functional relationship with the carnitine system [letter]? *Neurology* 1996; **46**(3): 851.

Beyer-Mears A, Diecke FP, Mistry K, Cruz E. Comparison of the effects of zopolrestat and sorbinil on lens myo-inositol influx. *Pharmacology* 1997; **54**(2): 76–83.

Beyer-Mears A, Mistry K, Diecke FP, Cruz E. Zopolrestat prevention of proteinuria, albuminuria and cataractogenesis in diabetes mellitus. *Pharmacology* 1996; **52**(5): 292–302.

Biro K, Jednakovits A, Kukorelli T, Hegedus E, Koranyi L. Bimoclomol (BRLP-42) ameliorates peripheral neuropathy in streptozotocin-induced diabetic rats. *Brain Res Bull* 1997; **44**(3): 259–263

Biro K, Palhalmi J, Toth AJ, Kukorelli T, Juhasz G. Bimoclomol improves early electrophysiological signs of retinopathy in diabetic rats. *Neuroreport* 1998; **9**(9): 2029–2033.

Buckingham RE, Al-Barazanji KA, Toseland CD, Slaughter M, Connor SC, West A, Bond B, Turner NC, Clapham JC. Peroxisome proliferator-activated receptor-gamma agonist, rosiglitazone, protects against nephropathy and pancreatic islet cell abnormalities in Zucker fatty rats. *Diabetes* 1998; **47**(8): 1326–1334.

Byrne MM, Goke B. Human studies with glucagon-like-peptide-1: potential of the gut hormone for clinical use. *Diabet Med* 1996; **13**(10): 854–860.

Clinical Investigator News. *Endocrinology.* July, 1998; 6(7): 8–10.

Connor SC, Hughes MG, Moore G, Lister CA, Smith SA. Antidiabetic efficacy of BRL 49653, a potent orally active insulin sensitizing agent, assessed in the C57BL/KsJ db/db diabetic mouse by non-invasive 1H NMR studies of urine. *J Pharm Pharmacol* 1997; **49**(3): 336–344.

Cotter MA, Cameron NE, Keegan A, Dines KC. Effects of acetyl- and proprionyl-L-carnitine on peripheral nerve function and vascular supply in experimental diabetes. *Metabolism* 1995; **44**(9): 1209–1214.

Deacon CF, Knudsen LB, Madsen K, Wiberg FC, Jacobsen O, Holst JJ. Dipeptidyl peptidase IV resistant analogues of glucagon-like peptide-1 which have extended metabolic stability and improved biological activity. *Diabetologia* 1998; **41**(3): 271–278.

De Palo E, Gatti R, Sicolo N, Padovan D, Vettor R, Federspil G. Plasma and urine free L-carnitine in human diabetes mellitus. *Acta Diabetol Lat* 1981; **18**(1): 91–95.

Drucker DJ. Glucagon-like peptides. *Diabetes* 1998; **47**(2): 159–169.

Dupre J, Behme MT, Hramiak IM, McFarlane P, Williamson MP, Zabel P, McDonald TJ. Glucagon-like peptide I reduces postprandial glycemic excursions in IDDM. *Diabetes* 1995; **44**(6): 626–630.

Edelstein D, Brownlee M. Aminoguanidine ameliorates albuminuria in diabetic hypertensive rats. *Diabetologia* 1992; **35**(1): 96–97.

el-Kebbi IM, Roser S, Pollet RJ. Regulation of glucose transport by pioglitazone in cultured muscle cells. *Metabolism* 1994; **43**(8): 953–958.

Enoki S, Mitsukawa T, Takemura J, Nakazato M, Aburaya J, Toshimori H, Matsukara S. Plasma islet amyloid polypeptide levels in obesity, impaired glucose tolerance, and non-insulin-dependent diabetes mellitus. *Diabetes Res Clin Pract* 1992; **15**(1): 97–102.

Fedele D, Giugliano D. Peripheral diabetic neuropathy. Current recommendations and future prospects for its prevention and management. *Drugs* 1997; **54**(3): 414–421.

Friedman EA, Distant DA, Fleishhacker JF, Boyd TA, Cartwright K. Aminoguanidine prolongs survival in azotemic-induced diabetic rats. *Am J Kidney Dis* 1997; **30**(2): 253–259.

Gedulin BR, Young AA. Hypoglycemia overrides amylin-mediated regulation of gastric emptying in rats. *Diabetes* 1998; **47**(1): 93–97.

Goke B, Fuder H, Wieckhorst G, Theiss U, Stridde E, Littke T, Kleist P, Arnold R, Lucker PW. Voglibose (AO-128) is an efficient alpha-glucosidase inhibitor and mobilizes the endogenous GLP-1 reserve. *Digestion* 1995; **56**(6): 493–501.

Gorio A, Di Giulio AM, Tenconi B, Donadoni L, Germani E, Bertelli A, Mantegazza P, Maccari F, Ramacci MT. Peptide alterations in autonomic diabetic neuropathy prevented by acetyl-L-carnitine. *Int J Clin Pharmacol Res* 1992; **12**(5–6): 225–230.

Gutniak MK, Larsson H, Heiber SJ, Juneskans OT, Holst JJ, Ahren B. Potential therapeutic levels of glucagon-like peptide I achieved in humans by a buccal tablet. *Diabetes Care* 1996; **19**(8): 843–848.

Gutniak MK, Larsson H, Sanders SW, Juneskans O, Holst JJ, Ahren B. GLP-1 tablet in type 2 diabetes in fasting and postprandial conditions. *Diabetes Care* 1997; **20**(12): 1874–1879.

Hammes HP, Brownlee M, Edelstein D, Saleck M, Martin S, Federlin K. Aminoguanidine inhibits the development of accelerated diabetic retinopathy in the spontaneous hypertensive rat. *Diabetologia* 1994; **37**(1): 32–35.

Hammes HP, Martin S, Federlin K, Geisen K, Brownlee M. Aminoguanidine treatment inhibits the development of experimental diabetic retinopathy. *Proc Natl Acad Sci USA* 1991; **88**(24): 11555–11558.

Hammes HP, Strodter D, Weiss A, Bretzel RG, Federlin K, Brownlee M. Secondary intervention with aminoguanidine retards the progression of diabetic retinopathy in the rat model. *Diabetologia* 1995; **38**(6): 656–660.

Ido Y, McHowat J, Chang KC, Arrigoni-Martelli E, Orfalian Z, Kilo C, Corr PB, Williamson JR. Neural dysfunction and metabolic imbalances in diabetic rats. Prevention by acetyl-L-carnitine. *Diabetes* 1994; **43**(12): 1469–1477.

Kanamaru M, Uematsu T, Nagashima S, Mizuno A, Terakawa M, Sugiyama A Nakashima M. Aldose reductase inhibitory and uricosuric activities of FK366 in healthy volunteers. *J Clin Pharmacol* 1993; **33**(11): 1122–1131.

Kobatake T, Matsuzawa Y, Tokunaga K, Fujioka S, Kawamoto T, Keno Y, Inui Y, Okada H, Matsuo T, Tarui S. Metabolic improvements associated with a reduction of abdominal visceral fat caused by a new alpha-glucosidase inhibitor, AO-128, in Zucker fatty rats. *Int J Obes* 1989; **13**(2): 147–154.

Koda JE, Fineman M, Rink TJ, Dailey GE, Muchmore DB, Linarelli LG. Amylin concentrations and glucose control. *Lancet* 1992; **339**: 1179–1180.

Kolterman OG, Gottlieb A, Moyses C, Colburn W. Reduction of postprandial hyperglycemia in subjects with IDDM by intravenous infusion of AC137, a human amylin analogue. *Diabetes Care* 1995; **18**(8): 1179–1182.

Kolterman OG, Schwartz S, Corder C, Levy B, Klaff L, Peterson J, Gottlieb A. Effect of 14 days' subcutaneous administration of the human amylin analogue, pramlintide (AC137), on an intravenous insulin challenge and response to a standard liquid meal in patients with

IDDM. *Diabetologia* 1996; **39**(4): 492–499.

Kong MF, King P, Macdonald IA, Stubbs TA, Perkins AC, Blackshaw PE, Moyses C, Tattersall RB. Infusion of pramlintide, a human amylin analogue, delays gastric emptying in men with IDDM. *Diabetologia* 1997; **40**(1): 82–88.

Kong MF, Stubbs TA, King P, Macdonald IA, Lambourne JE, Blackshaw PE, Perkins AC, Tattersall RB. The effect of single doses of pramlintide on gastric emptying of two meals in men with IDDM. *Diabetologia* 1998; **41**(5): 577–583.

Makita Z, Vlassara H, Rayfield E, Cartwright K, Friedman E, Rodby R, Cerami A, Bucala R. Hemoglobin-AGE: a circulating marker of advanced glycosylation. *Science* 1992; **258**(5082): 651–653.

Marzo A, Corsico N, Cardace G, Morabito E. Effect of acetyl-l-carnitine treatment on the levels of levocarnitine and its derivatives in streptozotocin-diabetic rats. *Arzneimittelforschung* 1993; **43**(3): 339–342.

Matsumoto K, Yano M, Miyake S, Ueki Y, Yamaguchi Y, Akazawa S, Tominaga Y. Effects of voglibose on glycemic excursions, insulin secretion, and insulin sensitivity in non-insulin-treated NIDDM patients. *Diabetes Care* 1998; **21**(2): 256–260.

Matsuo T, Odaka H, Ikeda H. Effect of an intestinal disaccharidase inhibitor (AO-129) on obesity and diabetes. *Am J Clin Nutr* 1992; **55**(1 Suppl): 314S–317S.

Morabito E, Serafini S, Corsico N, Martelli EA. Acetyl-l-carnitine effect of nerve conduction velocity in streptozotocin-diabetic rats. *Arzneimittelforschung* 1993; **43**(3): 343–346.

Mylari BL, Larson ER, Beyer TA, Zembrowski WJ, Aldinger CE, Dee MF, Siegel TW, Singleton DH. Novel, potent aldose reductase inhibitors: 3,4-dihydro-4-oxo-3-[[5-(trifluoromethyl)-2-benzotheiazolyl]methol]-1-phthalazineacetic acid (zopolrestat) and congeners. *J Med Chem* 1991; **34**(1): 108–122.

Nathan DM, Schreiber E, Fogel H, Mojsov S, Habener JF. Insulinotropic action of glucagon-like peptide-I-(7–37) in diabetic and nondiabetic subjects. *Diabetes Care* 1992; **15**(2): 270–276.

Nauck MA, Sauerwald A, Ritzel R, Holst JJ, Schmiegel W. Influence of glucagon-like peptide 1 on fasting glycemia in type 2 diabetic patients treated with insulin after sulfonylurea secondary failure. *Diabetes Care* 1998b; **21**(11): 1925–1931.

Nauck MA, Weber I, Bach I, Richter S, Orsakov C, Holst JJ, Schmiegel W. Normalization of fasting glycaemia by intravenous GLP-1 ([7–36 amide] or [7–37]) in type 2 diabetic patients. *Diabet Med* 1998a; **15**(11): 937–945.

Nauck MA, Wollschläger D, Werner J, Holst J, Ørskov C, Creutzfeldt W, Willms B. Effects of subcutaneous glucagon-like peptide 1 (GLP-1[7-36 amide]) in patients with NIDDM. *Diabetologia* 1996; **39**: 1546–1553.

Oakes ND, Camilleri S, Furler SM, Chisholm DJ, Kraegen EW. The insulin sensitizer, BRL 49653, reduces systemic fatty acid supply and utilization and tissue lipid availability in the rat. *Metabolism* 1997; **46**(8): 935–942.

Oakes ND, Kennedy CJ, Jenkins AB, Laybutt DR, Chisholm DJ, Kraegen EW. A new antidiabetic agent, BRL 49653, reduces lipid availability and improves insulin action and glucoregulation in the rat. *Diabetes* 1994; **43**(10): 1203–1210.

Okada S, Ishii K, Hamada H, Tanokuchi S, Ichiki K, Ota Z. The effect of an α-glucosidase inhibitor and insulin on glucose metabolism and lipid profiles in non-insulin-dependent diabetes mellitus. *J Int Med Res* 1996a; **24**: 438–447.

Okada S, Ishii K, Hamada H, Tanokuchi S, Ichiki K, Ota Z. The effect of a very low dose of tolbutamide combined with an α-glucosidase inhibitor in non-insulin-dependent diabetes mellitus. *J Int Med Res* 1996b; **24**: 433–437.

Onofrj M, Fulgente T, Melchionda D, Marchionni A, Tomasello F, Salpietro FM, Alafaci C, De Sanctis E, Pennisi G, Bella R, et al. L-acetylcarnitine as a new therapeutic approach for peripheral neuropathies with pain. *Int J Clin Pharmacol Res* 1995; **15**(1): 9–15.

Panagiotopoulos S, O'Brien RC, Bucala R, Cooper ME, Jerums G. Aminoguanidine has an anti-atherogenic effect in the cholesterol-fed rabbit. *Atherosclerosis* 1998; **136**(1): 125–131.

The Pink Sheet. Pfizer inhaled insulin to enter phase III in mid-1998, firm tells analysts: aldose reductase inhibitor Alond phase II trials show effect on nerve conduction. November 3, 1998, p. 8.

Quatraro A, Roca P, Donzella C, Acampora R, Marfella R, Giugliano D. Acetyl-L-carnitine for symptomatic diabetic neuropathy [letter]. *Diabetologia* 1995; **38**(1): 123.

Ramasamy R, Oates PJ, Schaefer S. Aldose reductase inhibition protects diabetic and nondiabetic rat hearts from ischemic injury. *Diabetes* 1997; **46**(2): 292–300.

Ritzel R, Orskov C, Holst JJ, Nauck MA. Pharmacokinetic, insulinotropic, and glucagonostatic properties of GLP-1 [7–36 amide] after subcutaneous injection in healthy volunteers. Dose-response relationships. *Diabetologia* 1995; **38**(6): 720–725.

Scherbaum WA. The role of amylin in the physiology of glycemic control. *Exp Clin Endocrinol Diabetes* 1998; **106**(2): 97–102.

Scrip No. 2320. Side effects with Alteon's pimagedine. March 25, 1998, p. 24.

Scrip No. 2322. Antidiabetic ADRs in Japan. April 1, 1998, p. 19.

Scrip No. 2338/39. Takeda/Lilly tie up on pioglitazone. May 27/29, 1998, p. 17.

Scrip No. 2345. SB buoyant on rosiglitazone Phase III data. June 19, 1998, p. 19.

Scrip No. 2351. Clinical trials update. July 10, 1998, p. 24.

Scrip No. 2382. Amylin stock drops 77% on pramlintide results. October 28, 1998, p. 20.

Scrip No. 2387. Pfizer to launch "new wave" of drugs. November 13, 1998, p. 12.

Scrip No. 2407. Additional data boosts confidence in pramlintide. January 29, 1999, p. 21.

Shinozaki K, Suzuki M, Ikebuchi M, Hirose J, Hara Y, Harano Y. Improvement of insulin sensitivity and dyslipidemia with a new α-glucosidase inhibitor, voglibose, in nondiabetic hyperinsulinemic subjects. *Metabolism* 1996; **45**(6): 731–737.

Solomon SS, Mishra SK, Cwik C, Rajanna B, Postlethwaite AE. Pioglitazone and metformin reverse insulin resistance induced by tumor necrosis factor-α in liver cells. *Horm Metab Res* 1997; **29**(8): 379–382.

Soneru IL, Khan T, Orfalian Z, Abraira C. Acetyl-l-carnitine effects on nerve conduction and glycemic regulation in experimental diabetes. *Endocr Res* 1997; **23**(1–2): 27–36.

Soulis T, Cooper ME, Sastra S, Thallas V, Panagiotopoulos S, Bjerrum OJ, Jerums G. Relative contributions of advanced glycation and nitric oxide synthase inhibition to aminoguanidine-mediated renoprotection in diabetic rats. *Diabetologia* 1997; **40**(10): 1141–1151.

Souza SC, Yamamoto MT, Franciosa MD, Greenberg AS. BRL 49653 blocks the lipolytic actions of tumor necrosis factor-alpha: a potential new insulin-sensitizing mechanism for thiazolidinediones. *Diabetes* 1998; **47**(4): 691–695.

Thompson RG, Pearson L, Kolterman OG. Effects of 4 weeks' administration of pramlintide, a human amylin analogue, on glycaemia control in patients with IDDM: effects on plasma glucose profiles and serum fructosamine concentrations. *Diabetologia* 1997b; **40**: 1278–1285.

Thompson RG, Pearson L, Schoenfeld SL, Kolterman OG, Pramlintide in Type 2 Diabetes Group. Pramlintide, a synthetic analog of human amylin, improves the metabolic profile of patients with type 2 diabetes using insulin. *Diabetes Care* 1998; **21**: 987–993.

Thompson RG, Peterson J, Gottlieb A, Mullane J. Effects of pramlintide, an analog of human amylin, on plasma glucose profiles in patients with IDDM. Results of a multicenter trial. *Diabetes* 1997a; **46**: 632–636.

Todd JF, Edwards CMB, Ghatei MA, Mather HM, Bloom SR. Subcutaneous glucagon-like peptide-1 improves postprandial glycaemic control over a 3-week period in patients with early type 2 diabetes. *Clin Sci (Colch)* 1998; **95**(3): 325–329.

Todd JF, Wilding JP, Edwards CM, Khan FA, Ghatei MA, Bloom SR. Glucagon-like peptide-1 (GLP-1): a trial of treatment in non-insulin-dependent diabetes mellitus. *Eur J Clin Invest* 1997; **27**(6): 533–536.

Towns R, Kostyo JL, Colca JR. Pioglitazone inhibits the diabetogenic action of growth hormone, but not its ability to promote growth. *Endocrinology* 1994; **134**(2): 608–613.

Vigh L, Literati PN, Horvath I, Torok Z, Balogh G, Glatz A, Kovacs E, Boros I, Ferdinandy P, Farkas B, Jaszlits L, Jednakovitz A, Koranyi L, Maresca B. Bimoclomol: a nontoxic, hydroxylamine derivative with stress protein-inducing activity and cytoprotective effects. *Nat Med* 1997; **3**(10): 1150–1154.

Yamasaki Y, Kawamori R, Wasada T, Sato A, Omori Y, Eguchi H, Tominaga M, Sasaki H,

Ikeda M, Kubota M, Ishida Y, Hozumi T, Baba S, Uehara M, Shichiri M, Kaneko T. Pioglitazone (AD-4833) ameliorates insulin resistance in patients with NIDDM. AD-4833 Glucose Clamp Study Group, Japan. *Tohuku J Exp Med* 1997; **183**(3): 173–183.

Yang CW, Yu CC, Ko YC, Huang CC. Aminoguanidine reduces glomerular inducible nitric oxide synthase (iNOS) and transforming growth factor-beta 1 (TGF-beta1) mRNA expression and diminishes glomerulosclerosis in NZB/W F1 mice. *Clin Exp Immunol* 1998; **113**(2): 258–264.

Young PW, Buckle DR, Cantello BC, Chapman H, Clapham JC, Coyle PJ, Haigh D, Hindley RM, Holder JC, Kallender H, Latter AJ, Lawrie KWM, Mossakoska D, Murphy GJ, Roxbee Cox L, Smith SA. Identification of high-affinity binding sites for the insulin sensitizer rosiglitazone (BRL-49653) in rodent and human adipocytes using a radioiodinated ligand for peroxisomal proliferator-activated receptor gamma. *J Pharmacol Exp Ther* 1998; **284**(2): 751–759.

Zimmerman GA, Meistrell M 3rd, Bloom O, Cockroft KM, Bianchi M, Risucci D, Broome J, Farmer P, Cerami A, Vlassara H, et al. Neurotoxicity of advanced glycation endproducts during focal stroke and neuroprotective effects of aminoguanidine. *Proc Natl Acad Sci USA* 1995; **92**(9): 3744–3748.

9

REGULATORY EXPECTATIONS FOR ANTIDIABETIC THERAPIES

The regulatory landscape for antidiabetic therapies has changed significantly over the past decade. Drug evaluation scientists at the Food and Drug Administration (FDA) have become increasingly active in the encouragement and guidance of drug developers. The FDA has used several advisory committee hearings to generate discussion about specific issues involved in the development of therapies for diabetes and related indications such as obesity. Symposia in these therapeutic areas more and more often involve the participation of regulators.

In order to respond to the explosion of interest in diabetes therapeutics following the report of the Diabetes Control and Complications Trial (DCCT), clinicians in the Division of Metabolic and Endocrine Drug Products intended to address a growing number of methodological issues associated with therapeutic development in diabetes. FDA recently prepared a draft guidance document on the evaluation of antidiabetic therapies. This early draft was discussed at a meeting of the Endocrinologic and Metabolic Drugs Advisory Committee of the FDA's Center for Drug Evaluation and Research on March 12, 1998. Although consensus was not reached for many of the points in the draft guidance, and different perspectives were apparent even among FDA participants, the issues raised at this meeting provide some insight into the future development of therapies designed to improve metabolic control and other aspects of diabetes. The issues of identifying and preventively treating those at high risk for developing diabetes was not addressed at the hearing or in the document, but these represent major opportunities for which guidance is urgently needed. The evaluation of therapies designed to treat or prevent diabetic complications was not addressed in this draft, but many of the topics are relevant for these compounds as well. The FDA is currently revising the guidance document, and another public hearing and/or publication for comment is expected before the middle of 2000. The FDA has issued draft or completed guidances for nearly all major therapeutic areas, including some related to diabetes (obesity, lipid-lowering, and osteoperosis therapies). These may be found on the Center for Drug Evaluation and Research Web page at www.cder.gov.

This chapter presents (with commentary) a summary of the guidance document and its advisory committee discussion. Current expectations for therapies aimed at diabetic complications are also provided.

PATIENT SELECTION AND DIAGNOSIS

Criteria for the clinical diagnosis of diabetes have recently been revised by the American Diabetes Association (ADA; American Diabetes Association, 1997). The new criteria reduce the cutoff point for fasting plasma glucose from ≥140 mg/dl to ≥126 mg/dl, and are expected to identify individuals with "early" type 2 diabetes. However, the ADA guidelines do not recommend pharmacological treatment for patients diagnosed only under these new criteria, raising questions as to whether these patients should be included in clinical trials of antidiabetic compounds. At the FDA Advisory Committee meeting, it was generally agreed that these patients should be allowed to participate in clinical trials, as the use of a baseline period including a diet and exercise regimen would be expected to screen out those patients for whom lifestyle modifications are adequate to achieve glycemic control.

Beyond these basic criteria, however, the appropriate patient population is dependent upon both the objective and the design of the study. Although a broad population is desirable from the standpoint of collecting generalizable results, there are ethical issues associated with the inclusion of certain patients in long-term, placebo-controlled studies. As substantial morbidity is associated with prolonged hyperglycemia, it is not acceptable to remove patients with severe hyperglycemia from adequate treatment and allow their condition to deteriorate on placebo over the course of a long-term study. Thus, placebo-controlled studies should generally be conducted in patients with relatively mild to moderate hyperglycemia. In the FDA's draft guidance, it is recommended that candidates have an initial HbA_{1c} level of 8.0% or less following a baseline period of intensified diet therapy; however, this issue is under some debate. Higher baseline HbA_{1c} values are likely to be acceptable for shorter studies, with more stringent criteria for longer studies. An alternative is to include individuals with higher HbA_{1c} levels, but to withdraw them from the study for lack of efficacy if their metabolic control has deteriorated after a certain amount of time. This would not be a suitable approach in situations in which the lack of treatment (placebo) is expected to be associated with a high withdrawal rate. A significant loss of patients from the placebo group would undermine the chief objective of placebo-controlled studies: to determine the treatment effect. The draft guidance suggests that for very short-term, placebo-controlled studies (4–6 weeks in duration), patients with a fasting plasma glucose level of up to 240 mg/dl may be enrolled.

Although patients naive to antidiabetic treatment are the most ideal population for placebo-controlled studies from an ethical standpoint, these patients are less common and relatively difficult to recruit in sufficient numbers. In addition, it is also important to evaluate a more diverse population of patients in clinical trials, as there may be substantial variability in response based on previous treatment history. For example, naive patients are most likely to respond to treatment, while patients who have a previous treatment failure are least likely to respond. In addition, newly diagnosed patients with mild hyperglycemia are likely to tolerate antidiabetic agents differently than moderate or severe diabetic patients with previous treatment failure, particularly with regard to the development of hypoglycemia. Furthermore, the overall treatment effect should be defined in the entire population for which the drug is intended. Providing only the treatment effect in a sensitive subset gives an inflated impression of the drug's effectiveness. Thus, efficacy should be formally assessed in subgroups defined by previous treatment and disease severity.

STUDY DESIGN

Placebo versus Active Controls

As with any indication, adequate and well-controlled studies are required to establish the efficacy and safety of antidiabetic compounds. However, some controversy related to the above discussion has grown over the use of placebo-controlled trials in the diabetic population. Although placebo-controlled studies are the gold standard for demonstrating efficacy, the consequences of prolonged hyperglycemia call into question the ethical acceptability of administering placebo on a long-term basis to diabetic individuals. The DCCT and, more recently, the United Kingdom Prospective Diabetes Study (UKPDS), have defined the benefits of glycemic control in preventing microvascular complications. Until these data became available, the estimate of the benefit-to-risk relationship of controlling hyperglycemia in type 2 patients with available therapies was far less favorable. The University Group Diabetes Program (UGDP), for example, suggested at best a marginally acceptable relationship (see Chapter 2). Today the benefits and risks for sulfonylurea and metformin therapies have largely been defined. This relatively new information has both stimulated the development of new therapies and made development more challenging because of the resulting placebo issue.

In discussions of the draft guidance, there was a general consensus that placebo-controlled studies are necessary in Phase II for the determination of efficacy. However, as noted in the previous section, the appropriate use of a placebo control is dependent upon several factors, including the population of patients under investigation, as well as the study duration. In patients with mild to moderate hyperglycemia, pivotal Phase II, placebo-controlled trials of 3–6 months duration are likely to provide an adequate assessment of efficacy without exposing patients to a harmful deterioration of metabolic control. A more stringent criterion for baseline HbA_{1c} would be required for a study lasting 6 months or more than for a shorter trial. In addition, dose-response properties of the compound should be determined in 2–4 week trials comparing placebo with at least three doses of the investigational compound. For all patients in these studies, diet and exercise should be emphasized prior to randomization and during the course of the study.

In contrast, the draft guidance stresses the use of active comparators in the design of larger, long-term (one year or more) Phase III trials. The draft itself suggested that such studies could be a primary basis for defining efficacy. However, ranking FDA officials stated at the hearing and elsewhere that the objective of these trials is to collect more comprehensive safety and tolerability data. The secondary objective is to provide supplementary information on efficacy. With an active control, it is possible to include a larger and more diverse range of diabetic patients, as well as a longer trial duration. Several types of trial designs may be appropriate at this stage (Figure 9.1). For example, rather than including a placebo arm, the investigational therapy might be evaluated alone and in combination with an active comparator, after an adequate baseline has been established with the active comparator. In studies with active comparators, the strategy of titrating doses to achieve roughly equivalent levels of glycemic control may allow for a more definitive comparison of relative safety and tolerability.

The selection of a suitable active control should be based on the characteristics of the population enrolled in the study and the underlying mechanism of the compound under

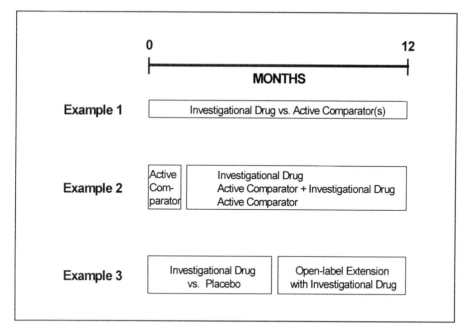

Figure 9.1 - Examples of potential designs in Phase III.

investigation. For example, sulfonylureas are not recommended for very mild patients, while α-glucosidase inhibitors may not be sufficiently potent for poorly controlled patients. Moreover, if the investigational compound is not associated with gastrointestinal adverse events, the use of an α-glucosidase inhibitor as a comparator may unblind the study. Finally, designs including a combination therapy arm are not appropriate for two compounds with similar mechanisms of action, unless the established therapy is used at the dose which achieves its maximum effect as monotherapy.

An illustrative example of a drug development program employing these principles is the New Drug Application for the meglitinide compound, repaglinide. The approval of repaglinide was based upon three relatively short-term, placebo-controlled studies as well as several long-term, active-controlled studies. Efficacy was shown in the short-term studies (maximum of 6 months in duration), in which repaglinide's treatment effect on HbA$_{1c}$ levels was demonstrated. In contrast, safety and tolerability were demonstrated in five one-year, active-controlled trials in which repaglinide and various sulfonylurea agents were titrated to achieve the same level of glycemic control, thus allowing a fair comparison of the safety of these therapies.

Durability of Effectiveness

Efficacy of therapies for glycemic control can be demonstrated in short periods of time – as little as one week for fasting plasma glucose and 12 weeks for HbA$_{1c}$. As diabetes is a life-long disease requiring chronic treatment, the durability of a drug's euglycemic effect is an important aspect of its clinical utility. The draft guidelines recommend that a sustained therapeutic effect on HbA_{1c} be demonstrated at 12 months. However, the difficulty of showing durability without a concurrent placebo control group is not adequately addressed in the draft. Active-controlled studies have been suggested as a means of evaluating the durability of efficacy, but this strategy is flawed in that it can only determine relative, not absolute, durability. Furthermore, a relatively large number of patients is required to establish the therapeutic equivalency of two compounds with similar efficacy. Results of studies using this approach are clouded by the effects of the natural progression of the disease. Open-label extension studies are another option, although this approach carries its own difficulties in interpretation. Confusion on this point was evident when this same advisory panel met again to consider the approvability of Ergoset™ (bromocriptine) for glycemic control of type 2 patients. The three placebo-controlled trials of Ergoset lasted for 6 months. At the end of each study, patients who had received Ergoset were briefly taken off therapy, and the therapy was then re-titrated. Placebo-treated patients were also allowed to go on treatment. Glycemic control of the pooled, treated patients continued to improve for about the next 6 months of therapy. With further passage of time and increasingly fewer patients, average HbA_{1c} drifted up to the extent that by the last observation point, these averages had returned to the baseline levels at the beginning of the controlled trials. Without a control group, it was impossible to determine the treatment effect beyond the control period. In all likelihood, the control of untreated patients would have continued to deteriorate more or less at the same rate observed during the controlled trial. Under this scenario, the treatment effect observed in the controlled trial would have been preserved with prolonged therapy. However, there was enough uncertainty about the durability of Ergoset's modest treatment effect among the advisory committee members that they voted to recommend non-approval. The lesson here is that durability of a treatment effect can only be determined if a concurrent control group is maintained for the entire period of interest. Since placebo treatment in most cases cannot ethically be justified for such durations, the only alternative is the use of an active treatment comparison. However, an active control comparison provides only a relative and not absolute indication of durability. Data from shorter-term studies may be sufficient if the treatment is associated with unusual benefits or is extremely safe.

Total Patient Exposure

Traditionally, the compilation of safety data from 1000 patient-years of exposure has been required by the FDA for the approval of antidiabetic therapies, with a certain subset of patients receiving the drug for one year or more. The new guidance suggests a total patient number of 2000 without fully specifying the distribution of patients across treatment durations. The International Conference of Harmonization of the Technical Requirements for Registration of Pharmaceuticals for Human Use (ICH) has issued a guidance on patient exposure for approval of drugs intended for the long-term treatment of non-life-threatening conditions. This document has become a guidance for the FDA and a regulation in Europe and Japan. The document specifies 300–600 patients exposed for six months and at least 100 patients for one year or longer. Greater numbers of patients may be necessary depending on the potential for rare adverse events, based on animal data or experience with compounds of the same class (e.g., lactic acidosis with metformin). The FDA will continue to require far more patient exposure for diabetes-related indications than specified by ICH. Whatever the minimum exposure requirement, it is clear that the bulk of patient exposure will come from large, Phase III, active-comparator trials; indeed, it is likely that nearly all of the patients exposed for at least one year will come from this category.

OUTCOME MEASURES

HbA$_{1c}$

The value of HbA$_{1c}$ as a primary efficacy measure in clinical trials of antidiabetic compounds is well established, as the results of the Diabetes Control and Complications Trial (DCCT) and United Kingdom Prospective Diabetes Study (UKPDS) convincingly demonstrated its utility as a surrogate marker for the development of microvascular complications in type 1 and type 2 diabetes (DCCT Research Group, 1993). However, the issue of how to determine "clinically significant" efficacy with regard to this measure is unresolved. Although the approval of acarbose was based on a sustained improvement of 0.7% in HbA$_{1c}$ levels, there is no clear minimum HbA$_{1c}$ treatment effect that can be considered clinically meaningful. This is largely due to the demonstration by the DCCT that even modest reductions in HbA$_{1c}$ levels can significantly reduce the occurrence of complications. Thus, smaller degrees of improvement may also be considered clinically significant. It is anticipated that the FDA will continue to determine approvability of agents for glycemic control on the basis of the overall benefit-to-risk relationship. This is despite the view of some FDA clinical reviewers that a minimal treatment effect of approximately 0.7 HbA$_{1c}$ units should be expected to qualify as an effective therapy.

An additional issue raised by the results of the DCCT is the expression of the *absolute* versus *percentage* change in HbA$_{1c}$ from baseline. Although the general practice has been to represent changes in HbA$_{1c}$ values as the absolute difference from baseline, it has been argued that the significance of the reduction in HbA$_{1c}$ is dependent upon the initial severity of the patient. In the DCCT trial, the percent reduction in HbA$_{1c}$ from baseline was proportional to the percent reduction in the risk of complications. Thus, it has been proposed that HbA$_{1c}$ data be presented as a percent change from baseline, in order to more easily correlate results with the predicted reduction of microvascular complications.

Another potential departure from general FDA policy suggested by the draft guidance is the requirement that new antidiabetic compounds demonstrate not only a significant reduction in HbA$_{1c}$ relative to the performance of a placebo group, but also an absolute reduction from the treated group's baseline values. The rationale for this prospective criteria is that a compound which maintains but does not lower hyperglycemia should not be approved for clinical use. However, an argument against this requirement is that diabetes is a progressive disease in which some deterioration is expected over a period of 3–12 months; thus, a therapy that slows or halts this natural progression should be considered efficacious. Furthermore, some decline in attention to diet, exercise, and medication compliance typically occurs over the course of a trial. The appropriate disposition of this bias is achieved in the classical definition of treatment effect, i.e., the difference between treatment and placebo group outcomes at endpoint, adjusted for any differences at baseline. The rationale for the position in the guidance is that the degree of deterioration observed during clinical trials in patients receiving placebo does not significantly represent the natural progression of the disease. Instead, this deterioration reflects the withdrawal from previous medication, the relaxation of diet and exercise regimens, or both. To some extent this issue is moot for mildly affected patients since they will typically show modest decline in glycemic control while on placebo. On the other hand, these patients are not reflective of the intended population. From an analytical perspective, the ideal approach is to randomize adequate numbers of patients, so that not only is the overall treatment effect a reasonable estimate of the therapy's performance in the real world, but outcomes in two or more disease severity subgroups can also be demonstrated. Although this issue remains unresolved, an adequate run-in period should be combined with an emphasis on diet and exercise in all patients throughout the study, in order to reduce the proportion of the treatment effect that is due to deterioration of control in the placebo group.

End-Organ Damage

The utility of HbA_{1c} as a primary outcome measure for antidiabetic compounds is based on its predictive value for the development of microvascular complications. Thus, if there is other evidence that a therapy significantly reduces the development of end-organ damage, this evidence clearly represents a primary outcome measure. However, the demonstration of a beneficial effect on long-term diabetic complications will most likely be based on surrogate markers that have yet to be determined. Some surrogate markers under consideration include biopsied nerve morphometry for neuropathy, retinal anatomic changes for retinopathy, and urinary albumin secretion for nephropathy. The selection of these outcome measures is becoming increasingly important, as a growing number of compounds are under development to directly treat or prevent the progression of diabetic complications. Clinical development issues for symptomatic therapies in diabetes are discussed in Chapter 10.

Hypoglycemia

As severe hypoglycemia is the rate-limiting obstacle to achieving euglycemia in patients on antidiabetic therapy, a reduction in the incidence of this adverse event (without a loss of glycemic control) is considered to be a primary outcome measure. However, the lack of a clear definition for severe hypoglycemia is problematic for assessment of this outcome in the context of clinical trials. In the DCCT, severe hypoglycemia was defined as an episode in which the patient required the assistance of another person, and that was associated with 1) a blood glucose level less than 50 mg/dl; or 2) reversal by oral carbohydrate, glucagon, or intravenous glucose (DCCT Research Group, 1997). The FDA draft guidance has suggested that similar criteria be instituted for clinical trials of antidiabetic therapies.

It should be noted that the DCCT was conducted in patients with type 1 diabetes, for whom severe hypoglycemia is more common. Under this definition, it is expected that the incidence of severe hypoglycemia will be relatively low in patients with type 2 diabetes, making it difficult to identify significant differences between therapies for the occurrence of this adverse event. For example, in the five large, active-controlled studies submitted for the approval of repaglinide, the results were suggestive of a decreased incidence of severe hypoglycemia with repaglinide therapy. These results did not reach statistical significance, potentially due to the low overall incidence of this adverse event. However, the documentation of milder episodes of hypoglycemia with home-glucose monitoring is less precise and reliable. Thus, although FDA recommends that lesser episodes of hypoglycemia be recorded during clinical trials as secondary efficacy criteria, these events are not considered to be adequate as primary outcome measures. It can be argued that a significant difference in simply those symptoms attributable to hypoglycemia has value for the patient. However, the FDA will respond that a truly meaningful difference in the performance of the treatments under comparison will be reflected in the criteria used in the DCCT.

Fasting and Average Plasma Glucose

Although HbA_{1c} is the universally accepted primary measure for the demonstration of efficacy, fasting and average plasma glucose levels have demonstrated a sufficiently high correlation with HbA_{1c} to serve as a secondary measure in pivotal trials, or a primary measure in short-term, dose-finding studies (Brewer et al., 1998; Kruseman et al., 1992). When used as a primary outcome measure, seven-point capillary blood glucose testing can be used to increase accuracy over home blood glucose monitors.

Other Outcome Measures

There are several additional factors that are not true outcome measures for efficacy, but may indicate potentially beneficial effects. For example, weight loss and an improvement in lipid profiles are desirable in type 2 diabetic patients, but are not considered to be evidence of efficacy unless accompanied by a reduction in hyperglycemia. In addition, the amelioration of hyperinsulinemia may have favorable effects on the development of macrovascular events. However, until this relationship is proven, it is not considered by the FDA as an outcome measure that, by itself, could justify an approval of an indication. Finally, a reduction in insulin dosage alone cannot be used to demonstrate efficacy, although the elimination of the need for insulin or a reduced need for frequent injections may be taken into consideration as a measure of efficacy.

DETERMINING LONG-TERM SAFETY

An important issue that has not yet been systematically addressed by regulatory agencies is the determination of long-term safety for chronic therapies. Although large, one-year, pivotal clinical trials are sufficient to characterize the overall safety and tolerability profile of an investigational compound, the ability to determine long-term safety or the risk of very rare adverse events is limited. For antidiabetic compounds, which are used chronically over the course of a life-long disease, this limitation can have serious consequences. For example, the association of lactic acidosis with phenformin therapy was revealed only after the drug had been marketed for nearly two decades, and reports of this adverse event had accumulated from physicians and patients. In addition, the results of the University Group Diabetes Program (UGDP) linking tolbutamide with an increase in cardiovascular mortality caused considerable concern that has only recently been addressed by the completion of the UKPDS. In other cases, data from pre-marketing or other trials may provide suggestive, but not conclusive, evidence of an association between the investigational drug and potentially serious adverse effects, raising questions regarding long-term safety that are not likely to be answered in one-year studies.

Drug safety issues that fall short of justifying non-approval or the removal of a therapy from the market have typically been addressed by the FDA with cautions or warnings in the labeling information. Such warnings have been used for antidiabetic compounds including metformin (lactic acidosis and cardiovascular mortality), the sulfonylureas (cardiovascular mortality), and troglitazone (liver toxicity). Although this is an easy mechanism for dealing with long-term safety issues, it does nothing but shift these difficult judgements to the prescribing physician.

The FDA has more recently addressed long-term safety issues for antidiabetic therapies by requiring post-approval studies designed to exclude significant adverse effects on survival. Several recent approvals of antidiabetic drugs (metformin, troglitazone, and repaglinide) have included requests by the FDA for the sponsors to perform these trials. In the case of repaglinide, for example, a weak signal was detected for excess cardiovascular events in comparison to sulfonylurea therapy in several active-controlled trials. This could only partially be explained by an imbalance in cardiac disease risk factors between treatment groups at baseline. Although the signal was not conclusive, the issue that it raised could only be resolved with an additional trial. Consequently, the sponsor company agreed to conduct post-approval a large, simple trial that will evaluate the relative risk of cardiovascular events in patients treated with repaglinide, a sulfonylurea, or insulin.

Government support for long-term outcome studies of antidiabetic therapies, chiefly from the National Institutes of Health (NIH), will continue and probably increase over the next decade. The importance of the DCCT and the UKPDS in galvanizing aggressive treatment of diabetes has been noticed by the U.S. Congress. Strong bipartisan support has developed for a variety of approaches aimed at reducing morbidity and mortality from this disease. Sponsorship of large outcome studies is a key strategy in these efforts. The National Heart, Lung, and Blood Institute, for example, is expected to announce a study designed to demonstrate the benefits of combining glycemic and hypertension control in patients with type 2 diabetes.

THE GLOBAL REGULATORY ENVIRONMENT

As clinical drug development has become an increasingly global process, the harmonization of requirements for the evaluation and approval of novel therapeutics has become an important goal. To achieve this goal, the International Conference on Harmonization of Technical Requirements for Registration of Pharmaceuticals for Human Use (ICH) has brought together six sponsors including the FDA's Center for Drug Evaluation and Research (CDER) and Center for Biologics Evaluation and Research (CBER), the European Federation of Pharmaceutical Industries Associations, the Japanese Ministry of Health and Welfare, and the Japanese Pharmaceutical Manufacturers Association to prepare guidelines that will encourage the standardization of various aspects of drug development.

The guidelines address numerous issues in four major areas: efficacy (human clinical trials), safety (animal pharmacology/toxicology), quality (manufacturing), and regulatory communication. To facilitate communication between regulatory agencies, a Medical Dictionary for Regulatory Activities that provides common terminology has recently been finalized. In addition, ICH has initiated the creation of a Common Technical Document for data presentation that may ultimately allow the submission of essentially the same information package to regulatory authorities in each of the participating regions.

While not all of the guidelines have been completed, the ICH initiative already appears to have made an impact on the pharmaceutical industry. In a survey of U.S., European, and

Japanese pharmaceutical companies by the Centre for Medicines Research (CMR) International, the majority of respondents indicated that ICH guidelines have increased some costs, but have also had a positive impact on the efficiency of clinical development programs (Scrip No. 2259, 1997).

CONCLUSIONS

The drug development process must balance the need for comprehensive safety and efficacy information with the need to bring effective novel therapies to the market in a timely manner. Moreover, the safety and rights of the patients participating in clinical trials must be protected. These concerns have created a number of methodological issues for the development of antidiabetic therapies, many of which are addressed in the recent FDA draft guidance on this topic. Consensus on these issues will be an instrumental step in clarifying regulatory expectations and enhancing the efficiency of drug development for this indication.

References

American Diabetes Association. Report of the expert committee on the diagnosis and classification of diabetes mellitus (committee report). *Diabetes Care* 1997; **20**: 1183–1197.

Brewer KW, Chase HP, Owen S, Garg SK. Slicing the pie. Correlating HbA$_{1c}$ values with average blood glucose values in a pie chart form. *Diabetes Care* 1998; **21**(2): 209–212.

DCCT Research Group. The effect of intensive treatment of diabetes on the development and progression of long-term complications in insulin-dependent diabetes mellitus. *N Eng J Med* 1993; **329**(14): 977–986.

DCCT Research Group. Hypoglycemia in the Diabetes Control and Complications Trial. *Diabetes* 1997; **46**: 271–286.

Kruseman AC, Mercelina L, Degenaar CP. Value of fasting blood glucose and serum fructosamine as a measure of diabetic control in non-insulin-dependent diabetes mellitus. *Horm Metab Res Suppl* 1992; **26**: 59–62.

McCombs JS. Pharmacoeconomics: what is it and where is it going? *AJH* 1998; **11**: 112S–119S.

National Diabetes Data Group. Classification and diagnosis of diabetes and other categories of glucose intolerance. *Diabetes* 1979; **28**: 1039–1057.

Scrip No. 2259. ICH efficacy guidelines push up costs. August 19, 1997, p. 12.

WHO Study Group on Diabetes Mellitus. *Diabetes mellitus: reports of a WHO Study Group*. Geneva: World Health Organization, 1985, p. 10–14.

10

METHODOLOGICAL CONSIDERATIONS: DIABETIC MICROVASCULAR COMPLICATIONS

The objective of this chapter is to present some of the methodological considerations associated with the assessment of diabetic complications caused by microangiopathy within the retina, peripheral nervous system, and kidney. Pertinent issues and assessment techniques related to the detection and measurement of diabetic retinopathy, neuropathy, and nephropathy will be reviewed, and recommendations for methodological procedures and analytic techniques are suggested that may be helpful in the implementation of controlled clinical trials designed to assess the efficacy of therapeutic agents for these complications.

DIABETIC RETINOPATHY

Microvascular complications of diabetes account for a significant degree of associated morbidity and mortality; as one of the most common complications of diabetes, retinopathy-associated visual loss is undoubtedly one of the most distressing for patients. The development of retinopathic complications is mediated by several important risk factors and moderator variables which influence both the prevalence and degree of diabetic microangiopathy expressed as retinopathy. The most important of these variables include duration of diabetes, the presence of nephropathy, hypertension, and glycemic control.

As noted in Chapter 2, the early stages of diabetic retinopathy are characterized by increases in capillary permeability and closures, as well as microaneurysms and retinal hemorrhages. These vascular manifestations can progress to a proliferative stage that is characterized by more severe hemorrhaging, scarring, and retinal detachment. Retinopathy tends to occur early in the diabetic disease process, and is typically the first detectable microvascular complication. The frequency of diabetic retinopathy also increases with the duration of illness. In fact, it has been estimated that nearly all patients with type 1 diabetes and approximately 60% of patients with type 2 diabetes will develop retinopathy after 20 years (Klein & Klein, 1997). As a result, diabetes remains a major cause of visual disability and blindness among active adults in economically-developed societies (Cunha-Vaz, 1998).

The presence of nephropathy and hypertension has also been implicated in the development of diabetic retinopathy. For example, Gilbert et al. (1998) reported that patients with type 1 diabetes with evidence of nephropathy may be at higher risk of developing diabetic retinopathy than patients who remain persistently normoalbuminuric. This contrast between groups was observed despite comparable long-term glycemic control and duration of diabetes. It has also been observed that retinal hemorrhaging and microaneurysms are relatively frequent in older populations who are not diabetic, and these visual abnormalities are significantly related to the presence and severity of hypertension (Yu et al., 1998). Thus, hypertension is a recognized risk factor in the development of visual impairment that is not specific to diabetes.

A convincing relationship between glycemic control and the development of diabetic retinopathy has been demonstrated in several studies. For example, in the Diabetes Control and Complications Trial (DCCT), examination of patients with type 1 diabetes (with no to moderate nonproliferative retinopathy) revealed a strong relationship between glycemic control and retinopathy. Though an early worsening of retinopathy was observed at the 6 and/or 12-month visits (13.1% of 711 patients assigned to intensive treatment and 7.6% of 728 patients assigned to conventional treatment), rates were roughly equivalent for both groups of patients (51% and 55%, respectively) by 18 months. With cumulative 8.5-year follow-up, those assigned to intensive glycemic control showed a 60% reduction in three- or more step progression of retinopathy compared with those on conventional therapy. These results indicate that the long-term benefits of intensive insulin treatment outweigh the risk of early worsening of retinopathic symptoms.

The timing of glycemic control may also be an important mediating variable in the relationship between glycemic control and the development of retinopathy. Danne et al. (1998) have hypothesized that long-term poor glycemic control, both before and after puberty, constitutes a major risk factor for the development of retinopathy. This group further suggested that HbA_{1c} levels during the first year of diabetes are related in an exponential, non-linear fashion to the later development of background retinopathy, in addition to other factors such as age at onset, puberty, lipids, blood pressure, genetic factors, and smoking, which are important independent contributors to diabetic retinopathy for individual patients. The notion of a "critical window" for the later development of diabetic complications has also been implicated in the development of diabetic neuropathy, in which poor glycemic control in the first few years after the onset of diabetes may be the crucial catalyst in the later development of neuropathy, regardless of subsequent efforts at glycemic control.

Some researchers have proposed that the protective effect of good glycemic control on retinopathy holds for both types of diabetes, and may extend across all ages and stages of retinopathy up to and including the severe nonproliferative and early proliferative stages (Davis, 1998). It has also been suggested that reducing elevated blood lipids and treating anemia may slow the progression of retinopathy. For example, for a patient with diabetes onset before age 50, a reduction of HbA_{1c} from 9% to 7% can result in a decrease from 2.6% to 0.3% in the lifetime risk for blindness secondary to retinopathy (Vijan et al., 1997). The same holds true for patients with an onset of diabetes at age 65. Their risk for blindness should decrease from 0.5% to <0.1%. However, it is important to note that individual predicted benefit depends upon the degree of glycemic control. Substantially greater benefit is seen when improvement occurs from poor to moderate glycemic control than from moderate to almost normal glycemic control.

Assessment of Diabetic Retinopathy

Early recognition provides the opportunity for expedient and effective treatment, and preservation of visual functioning. However, there are few agreed-upon measures to reliably evaluate the presence of diabetic retinopathy, and even fewer that allow for convenient, accurate, and reliable assessment of changes in diabetic retinopathy associated with various therapeutic agents. Some of the more promising methods for quantification of diabetic retinopathy include psychophysical methods, angiography, autofluoresence, electroretinography, Doppler imaging, and fundus photography.

Color Vision and Contrast Sensitivity

Jeddi et al. (1994) reported that various dependent measures of color vision and central field functioning were impaired in diabetic patients with no apparent diabetic retinopathy or with only background retinopathy. Color field deficits were observed in 57%, and visual field disturbances in 35%, of the cases. Importantly, color vision deficits preceded the appearance of angiographic diabetic retinopathy in approximately one half of the cases, and visual field disturbance predated actual retinopathy in approximately one third of the cases.

Color vision and contrast sensitivity testing have also been shown to effectively discriminate diabetic from non-diabetic subjects (Ewing et al., 1998). Moreover, the degree of impairment seen on these psychophysical measures may be associated with grade of diabetic retinopathy. Changes in contrast sensitivity have been reported in both children and adults with diabetes of short duration, and there is some preliminary evidence suggesting a relationship between contrast sensitivity and level of glycemic control (Ewing et al., 1998). Although a similar pattern is observed for color vision, a direct comparison of the two methods suggests that contrast sensitivity is a more specific and sensitive measure than color vision (Ewing et al., 1998). Contrast sensitivity measures may also reflect the integrity of foveal microcirculation in early diabetics with good visual acuity and no macular edema (Arend et al., 1997). This group reported that alterations in the perifoveal network were related to disturbances of visual function as measured by contrast sensitivity.

Autofluorescent Techniques

Autofluorescent techniques have also been shown to have some utility in the detection and measurement of diabetic retinopathy. For example, corneal and lens autofluoresence values measured by fluorophotometry in young type 1 diabetic patients without retinopathy were higher relative to control subjects (Ishiko et al., 1998). Lens fluorophotometry values were also significantly associated with duration of diabetes. Furthermore, corneal fluorophotometry values correlated with duration of diabetes and indices of metabolic control such as HbA_{1c} levels, suggesting that fluorophotometry measures may serve as reliable indicators of metabolic control. Importantly, these researchers reported that lens and corneal abnormalities were apparent before the appearance of overt diabetic retinopathy. This finding was also supported by Jeddi et al. (1994) who suggested that impairment on fluorescein angiography preceded actual damage of the fundus in 27% of cases in patients with no or background retinopathy, allowing for early treatment intervention that has been shown to result in less severe visual disturbance.

Electroretinography and Doppler Imaging

Focal electroretinography, which measures the functional integrity of the distal retina or the macula has also been proposed as a sensitive technique to identify and track the severity of diabetic retinopathy. In one such study, focal electroretinography measures were recorded by Deschenes et al. (1997) with a hand-held stimulator-ophthalmoscope in patients with type 2 diabetes. This group reported that implicit time and amplitude were significantly delayed and reduced in diabetic patients with retinopathy compared to control subjects. Additionally, implicit time and amplitude were associated with the duration of diabetes but not with HbA_{1c} levels. This group concluded that early macular degeneration in type 2 diabetic patients occurs before the appearance of overt diabetic retinopathy.

Another group of imaging techniques, referred to collectively as Doppler imaging, has also shown promise in the measurement of diabetic retinopathy. These techniques allow for two-dimensional anatomic imaging and measurement of blood flow velocities. It has been reported that patients with proliferative diabetic retinopathy have slower ocular perfusion velocities than control subjects, as assessed through color Doppler imaging techniques (Mendvil & Cuartero, 1996). Fujio et al. (1996) also supported the utility of a new laser Doppler instrument to measure retinal blood flow that is equipped with eye-tracking systems that maintain the laser beam on the retinal vessel at all times. This technique enables accurate measurement of patients with impaired visual acuity and poor fixation. This group reported that retinal flow was decreased in diabetic patients (even those without retinopathy) compared to control subjects, and that this was due to decreased retinal blood speed. This method also allows for the accurate quantification of retinal circulatory changes in retinal branch vessel occlusions.

Fundus Photography

However, the most widely used and accepted technique to assess the presence of diabetic retinopathy, which also allows for a reliable measure of change following treatment intervention, is fundus photography. Several objective methods are available. One such method proposed by Aldington et al. (1995) involves 45 degrees retinal photography and field grading carried out by a trained reader of color photographs. This method compared well to the standard of seven-field 30 degrees stereo photography, and detected retinal lesions in all cases detected by the standard method.

The standard method referred to above is also known as seven-standard field fundus photography. This method is considered to be the gold standard in the measurement of retinopathic changes and has been shown to be sensitive to treatment effects in both naturalistic and controlled clinical trials. In one such population study, Rajala et al. (1998) examined the fundus photographs of 790 subjects and found that 3.5% of subjects had mild retinopathic changes that were associated with higher fasting glucose levels. The prevalence of retinopathy was 10.2% in subjects with a fasting glucose of ≥6.1mmol/L.

Therefore, this method can be useful in discriminating patients at high risk for developing retinopathy.

However, it should be noted that this technique involves significant training and specialized equipment. Specifically, the use of a non-mydriatic fundus camera or a 30 degree Zeiss FF series fundus camera is required. In this technique, the seven standard fields of the fundus are obtained in stereo for each eye by a certified photographer. The seven fields are obtained in a standard sequence: disc (Field 1), macula (Field 2), temporal to macula (Field 3), superior temporal (Field 4), superior nasal (Field 6), inferior temporal (Field 5), and inferior nasal (Field 7).

In taking stereo photographs, careful attention must be paid to a variety of factors. The following procedure for taking stereo fundus photographs (developed by Allen, 1964) addresses these factors and helps to ensure accurate assessment of retinopathy. First, the pupil should be well dilated, preferably 6 mm or more, and the cornea should be undisturbed by prior examination with a diagnostic contact lens. The patient should be rested and not exhausted by too many other examinations or annoyed by long waiting, and the photographer should have adequate time to work carefully. A stereoscopic viewer for examining stereo fundus photographs is required, so that the photographer can critically examine his or her work and make appropriate corrections in technique. An Allen stereo separator or manual lateral movement of the camera may be used to obtain the required nonsimultaneous stereo. A non-stereo fundus reflex photograph should be taken in addition to those required of the seven standard fields. In addition to documenting the condition of the lens, the fundus reflex photograph allows graders to take opacities of the media into consideration when reviewing photographic quality. The fixation target may be used to direct the subject's gaze in the primary (straight ahead) position, so that the disc does not appear – in actual practice, the approach to the quantification and tracking of retinopathy through fundus photography is associated with considerable challenges in a multicenter trial environment, largely due to the coordination of patient availability with that of clinical and photographic personnel.

Regulatory Perspective

The major attempt at developing a medical therapy for retinopathy ended when the Sorbinil Retinopathy Study (SRT) failed to demonstrate a treatment effect of this aldose reductase inhibitor (ARI; The Sorbinil Retinopathy Trial Research Group, 1990). In all likelihood, the doses tried did not provide sufficient enzyme inhibition to allow a conclusive test of the hypothesis. Should more potent ARIs prove effective in neuropathy trials, this approach for retinopathy might be tried again.

The most important development since SRT is the accumulation of conclusive evidence that laser therapy is highly effective in preserving vision in patients with retinopathy. This surgical intervention is effective for the two major vision-threatening manifestations of retinopathy, macular edema and proliferative retinopathy. Though both retinopathic pathways are ultimately the result of impaired glycemic control and may develop concurrently, each has distinctive mechanisms. Macular edema appears to result from leaky retinal vessels. Proliferative retinopathy seems to be driven by growth factor-mediated signals from ischemic retinal tissue. Focal laser therapy is indicated for patients with macular edema, and pan-retinal laser therapy is indicated for treatment of pre-proliferative retinal changes. The proven effectiveness of laser therapy has posed a possible difficulty concerning endpoints for the development of anti-retinopathy medical therapies.

A debate about this issue within the FDA led to an advisory committee in January, 1998. Opthalmologic reviewers at the FDA had previously expressed the view that visual function would be the only acceptable outcome on which drug approvals could be based. Other evaluators concluded that this would be unreasonable because laser intervention had greatly reduced the event rate for visual loss. The diagram in Figure 10.1 illustrates the problem for developing medical therapy. Patients become eligible for laser therapy when they develop either moderate to severe non-proliferative retinopathy (NPR) or non-clinically significant macular edema (NSME). Laser intervention dramatically reduces the progression of patients into the more advanced categories of proliferative retinopathy (PR) and clinically significant macular edema (CSME). As shown by the Diabetic Retinopathy Study (DRS; The Diabetic Retinopathy Study Group, 1976, 1978) and the Early Treatment Diabetic Retinopathy Study (ETDRS; Early Treatment Diabetic Retinopathy Study, 1987), patients treated with laser therapy for both NPR and NSME have a much slower rate of visual function loss than untreated patients.

Because of the greatly reduced progression to visual loss that results after laser intervention, clinical trials of medical therapy would require as many as 20,000 NPR/NSME patients per treatment group for 3-4 years in order to show an effect on visual function. Clearly such trials would not be economically viable. If laser therapy is so effective, it might seem that laser therapy has obviated the need for medical therapy. This is not the case because laser therapy itself leads to some visual loss and other opthalmic complications. Laser therapy is also expensive, and long term outcomes (that is, greater than 10 years) following laser therapy are not known.

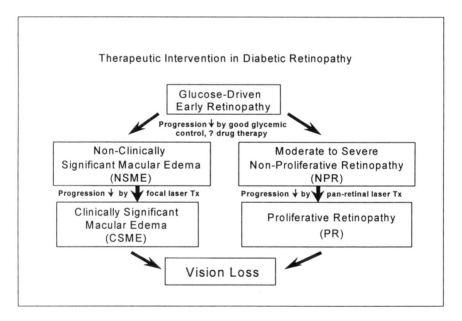

Figure 10.1 – Schematic of therapeutic options for diabetic retinopathy.

There are several candidate outcomes for evaluating medical therapy. Laser intervention itself would appear to be a reasonable surrogate. However, the timing of laser intervention is not fully standardized, thus increasing the variability of this measure. Ultimately the FDA advisory committee decided that the most reasonable endpoint would be progression to PR/CSME.

DIABETIC NEUROPATHY

Diabetic neuropathy, ranging from reversible mononeuropathies to irreversible and progressive autonomic neuropathy, is a serious and all-too-common complication of patients suffering from diabetes. Neuropathy has been associated with considerable morbidity in the form of painful polyneuropathy and neuropathic ulceration, and mortality from autonomic neuropathy. In fact, it is estimated that in 50–80% of cases, microvascular or macrovascular complications account for death.

Diabetic microangiopathy affects the capillaries and pre-capillary arterioles, and these vascular changes predispose patients to neuropathy and retinopathy. The actual causes of these vascular changes remain unknown; however, several common pathophysiological mechanisms such as basal membrane alterations and changes in barrier function affect the glomerular filters and microvasculature of the eyes and nerves. These vascular changes reduce blood flow, which leads to hypoxia. This in turn may lead to neuronal disruption manifested by reduced nerve conduction velocity (NCV).

Unlike other types of peripheral neuropathy, which tend to affect large diameter nerve fibers, diabetic neuropathy involves small myelinated and non-myelinated nerves, and is therefore considered to be a "length-dependent" distal axonopathy. Bilateral sensory or sensorimotor polyneuropathy is the most common clinical manifestation of diabetic neuropathy. Clinical signs and symptoms of diabetic neuropathy include paresthesia, reduced perception of temperature and vibration, and neuropathic pain. As the disease progresses, larger numbers of small and large fiber axons are damaged, resulting in both motor and sensory disturbances. Both type 1 and type 2 diabetic patients have been shown to exhibit motor nerve conduction abnormalities that may be related to disease duration (Gregersen, 1967). Furthermore, autonomic neuropathy can result in further dysfunction including gastric atony/paresis, bladder atony, impotence, and cardiovascular disturbances. In an effort to avoid such manifestations of diabetic neuropathy, it is essential to ensure accurate detection of early signs and symptoms as soon as possible.

Assessment Strategies in Diabetic Neuropathy

The epidemiology and natural history of diabetic neuropathy is uncertain, largely due to confusion created by a lack of adequate and well-accepted outcome measures. This may stem partially from the myriad and often non-standardized assessment techniques utilized in prior studies of diabetic neuropathy. It is therefore difficult to determine which or how many measurement techniques should be utilized when examining the impact of treatment on diabetic complications. This section will review several measures that have gained some recognition and acceptance in recent controlled clinical trials.

As expected, electrophysiological measures remain the preferred method of assessment in traditional nerve conduction studies, as they are a principal objective measure of functional integrity in diabetic sensorimotor neuropathy (Dyck, 1991; DCCT Research Group, 1993). In general, electrophysiological examinations involve recording the conduction velocity and amplitude for multiple nerves, both sensory and motor. These measures are sensitive and specific for polyneuropathy and represent accepted surrogate endpoints for clinical outcomes. However, even a comprehensive battery examines only a portion of functional neurons, and maximal conduction velocity reflects activity in only the fastest myelinated fibers. Thus, significant changes in small axons, the type most directly affected in diabetes, remain unmeasured in protocols that incorporate conduction velocity measurements alone. Complementary tests should also be used to maximize the chance of detecting a treatment effect.

In addition to traditional electrophysiological measures, comprehensive clinical neurological evaluations can help to characterize patients at baseline and to monitor disease severity throughout treatment. Quantitative sensory testing, as with the Computer-Assisted Sensory Evaluation system, version IV (CASE-IV; Dyck et al., 1978; Guy et al., 1985), is useful as a sensitive and specific marker of peripheral nerve dysfunction. Quantitative autonomic examination, as measured by variation in R-R interval on ECG during respiration (Pfeiffer et al., 1987), is an accepted clinical outcome. Urinary truncated nerve growth factor receptor, as a marker of peripheral nerve injury and regeneration, may be useful for exploratory studies (Hruska et al., 1993). As pain is a common feature associated with diabetic neuropathy, the potential for an associated symptomatic effect should also be assessed as a secondary measure. However, improvement in pain and paresthesias alone do not prove a positive therapeutic effect on the neuropathic process, but also can reflect a simple anesthetic effect or even a worsening of the neuropathy.

Nerve morphometry as determined by sural nerve biopsies has been used as a primary efficacy outcome in a few clinical studies. This approach is unlikely to be used in the future because the procedure is invasive, cannot be repeated more than twice, is not validated for reproducibility or relevance in diabetic neuropathy, and presents some risk for the development of a fixed sensory deficit and other complications. Cutaneous biopsies have been suggested as a relatively non-invasive method for assessing peripheral nerve morphology, but the experimental nature of this procedure and the related technical encumbrances render this procedure unfeasible in many studies (Kennedy & Wendelschafer-Crabb, 1994). Nerve biopsy continues to be useful, and in some cases necessary, to ensure penetration of the drug into the nerve and/or to confirm desired activity (e.g., aldose reductase inhibition). Only a small number of patient biopsies are necessary for achieving these objectives.

Electrophysiological Measures

Peroneal motor nerve conduction, obtained using standard methods employed in the electromyography (EMG) laboratory, remains one of the most utilized primary dependent measures for the assessment of treatment effects in controlled clinical trials of diabetic neuropathy. Specific measurements should include the distance between stimulation sites and the distance between the distal stimulation site and the recording site. The amplitude and the distal latency should be measured, and the NCV calculated.

The peroneal maximum motor nerve conduction velocity (MNCV), amplitude, and distal latency should be evaluated using the guidelines below:

- The distance between the recording and stimulating electrodes should be standardized at 9.0 cm measured in a straight line with calipers.

- Supramaximal stimulation should be approached by gradually increasing the amount of voltage or current until no further increase in the evoked compound muscle action potential is obtained, then by increasing the stimulus by another 10–20% and recording the response.

- Surface temperature should be >32°C (34°C is recommended) for 10 minutes prior to initiation of nerve conduction studies.

An abnormality in motor nerve conduction may be considered to be present if there is an abnormality in the conduction velocity, amplitude, and/or distal latency of the peroneal motor nerve. Abnormality can be defined as an amplitude of ≤2.0 mv, a conduction velocity of ≤45 m/s or a distal latency ≤6.5 ms.

Sural sensory NCV may also be obtained as a secondary outcome measure using standard methods as described above for the peroneal nerve.

The amplitude, conduction velocity, and distal latency of the median sensory and sural nerves can be evaluated using the guidelines below:

- All stimulations should be antidromic and percutaneous with a 30 mm separation between surface pick-up and reference electrodes.

- The cathode should be distal to the anode.

- Distal latency should be measured as time-to-negative peak.

- Amplitude should be measured from baseline to negative peak.

- Sural nerve stimulation should be 14 cm proximal to the recording electrode for the basic study and 7 and 21 cm for determining conduction velocity.

- Median sensory stimulation should be 14 cm proximal to the recording electrode (wrist-index finger). Ring electrodes should be placed over the index finger with 30 mm of separation between the recording and reference electrodes.

- Skin temperatures using an infrared lamp should be maintained at 34°C for 10 minutes prior to initiation of nerve conduction studies.

An abnormality in sensory nerve conduction may be considered to be present if there is an abnormality in the conduction velocity, amplitude, and/or distal latency of either nerve. For amplitude these are defined as ≤ 13μv for the median sensory nerve (wrist-index) and 0 μv for the sural nerve. Abnormalities in conduction velocity are defined as ≤54 m/s and ≤43 m/s for the median and sural nerves, respectively. Finally, abnormalities for distal latency are defined as ≤3.6 ms and ≤4.4 ms for the median and sural nerves, respectively.

Clinical Assessments

Mayo Clinic Classification for Diabetic Peripheral Neuropathy (Dyck, 1988)

This staging system is based on the Mayo Clinic classification for diabetic peripheral neuropathy, also called the Dyck criteria. Patients are categorized from stage 0 (no symptoms and fewer than two abnormalities on electrodiagnostic clinical tests) through stage III (a disabling symptomatic neuropathy with at least two abnormalities on electrodiagnostic and clinical examination). Staging requires a series of tests, including nerve conduction studies, a Neuropathy Disability Score (NDS), quantitative sensory testing (using the CASE-IV), and a Neuropathy Symptom Score (NSS), as well as a general clinical evaluation.

Quantitative Sensory Tests: Computer-Assisted Sensory Evaluation, Version IV (CASE-IV) (Adapted from Dyck et al., 1978)

The components of the testing system include the following: stimulator assemblies, electromechanical translator, electronic controller, computer, visual numerical display, patient response key, data storage disk, and printer. The touch pressure and vibration systems use components with separate stimulator assemblies. The thermal stimulator system does not include an electromechanical translator and has a separate stimulator assembly. In a recommended procedure, the patient is tested in a separate room within the laboratory, which is shielded from sound. The patient sits in a chair that includes a hydraulic scissors platform so that the finger or toe can be positioned. A videotape which describes the purpose of the procedure and the possibility of associated discomfort may be shown to the patient. The patient may have a trial session with the examiner to enhance familiarity with the procedures, and the examiner reinforces the instructions through a verbal description. Graded and reproducible cold detection threshold, vibratory threshold, and thermal pain discrimination stimuli are delivered to the patient. Responses are recorded, stored, and plotted graphically. In addition, a heat pain analogue scale is completed. Comparisons to the normal responses of demographically-matched control subjects from published databases provide the bases for defining abnormalities. Identical, predetermined testing algorithms are applied to each patient.

Neuropathy Disability Score (NDS; Dyck et al., 1980)

The NDS, administered by a physician or other trained clinician, assesses the severity of motor and sensory autonomic deficits. Individual items are scored on a scale of 0 to 4 (0 for no deficit through 4 for complete absence of function or severest deficit) and all item scores are summed. Abnormality is defined as a total score greater than 6. The NDS has been shown to be correlated with age and HbA_{1c} levels (Shaw et al., 1998). These factors accounted for 31% of the total variance of the NDS in patients with type 1 diabetes. When considered in conjunction with motor condition velocity, the NDS has been shown to have good prognostic validity in type 1 diabetes (Negrin et al., 1995).

Neuropathy Symptom Score (NSS; Dyck, 1980)

The NSS assesses neurological symptoms as reported by the patient. The assessment should be performed by a neurologist experienced in the evaluation of peripheral neuropathy. All symptoms are essentially descriptions volunteered by the patient through the use of non-directive inquiry. Positive responses are verified by an additional unstructured interview. Although analyses of symptoms can be based upon individual items, identified subsets include motor, sensory, and autonomic symptoms.

Quality of Life (QOL) and Mood Assessments

Social, psychological, and physical aspects all contribute to patients overall quality of life (QOL). Rose et al. (1998) reported that the overall QOL in diabetic patients appears to be somewhat better than in other chronically ill patients. As a result, they reported that physical complaints are assigned relatively lower weightings in diabetic patients than in other chronically ill patients with inflammatory bowel disease or chronic hepatitis. Given this, they hypothesized that the various components involved in overall QOL assessments (such as social, psychological and physical elements) should receive differential weightings, inferring that a simple, additive summary score for QOL may be invalid. It is important to note that coping behavior and various personality traits covaried with these QOL measures. Thus, psychological variables may have greater significance than the existence of secondary illnesses in QOL assessment and should be assessed in a systematic manner.

Sickness Impact Profile (SIP; Bergner et al., 1981)

The SIP is a patient-based QOL measure in which patients report health-related dysfunction on the day of the interview. It includes 12 different categories divided into three dimensions: a physical dimension that assesses ambulation, mobility, body care, and movement; a psychosocial dimension that assesses social interaction, alertness, emotional behavior, and communication; and an overall score that incorporates these categories with additional categories, including work, eating, sleep and rest, home management, and recreation and pastimes. Overall and dimension scores range from 0 to 100, with 100 representing maximal dysfunction. An increase in SIP score from baseline indicates more severe self-perceived sickness, while a decrease denotes improvement. One benefit of utilizing the SIP is that information can be obtained by centrally-located trained interviewers who are in direct contact with patients; the data ascertainment procedures do not have to involve site personnel. Thus, the SIP can provide a truly independent (from sponsor and site) evaluation of patient-perceived illness in diabetes.

Medical Outcomes Study Short-Form 36-item Health Survey (SF-36; Medical Outcomes Trust, 1992)

This is a general health questionnaire used to assess pain and other conditions during the past 4 weeks. It is used in international studies, as it allows data extrapolation across diseases and countries. Specifically, this form is designed to assess eight aspects of health, ranging from physical limitations to general perceptions of vitality and mental well-being. The SF-36 has shown some utility in the assessment of improvement of QOL in patients with upper gastrointestinal symptoms of diabetic gastroparesis. Silvers et al. (1998) reported that patients who responded to domperidone exhibited significant improvements in SF-36 physical and mental component summary scores. However, patients in the placebo group exhibited a significant deterioration in the physical component summary score compared with patients in the active treatment group. Interestingly, researchers such as Wienberger et al. (1994) have failed to find a relationship between various measures of glycemic control and overall QOL as assessed by the SF-36. These researchers proposed that the lack of relationship between these two variables might help explain the high noncompliance rates observed in patients on complex diabetic regimens. This implies that it may be difficult to achieve good glycemic control in patients who do not perceive a significant benefit in QOL derived from complex treatment regimens.

Profile of Mood States (POMS; McNair et al., 1971)

The POMS, designed to assess transient, distinct mood states, is composed of 65 adjectives rated by subjects on a 5-point scale ranging from 0 (not at all) to 4 (extremely). The various mood states can be characterized as follows: Tension-Anxiety, Depression-Dejection, Anger-Hostility, Fatigue-Inertia, Vigor-Activity, and Confusion-Bewilderment. In an examination of the relationship between hypoglycemia and mood, Merbis et al. (1996) reported that the progression of hypoglycemia negatively alters overall mood. They reported that type 1 diabetic patients characterized by high hostility scores on the Symptom Checklist-90 (SCL-90) were more prone to experience an increase in anger on the POMS during hypoglycemia. Thus, the accurate assessment of emotional states may vary according to glycemic control.

Special Assessment Procedures

Truncated Nerve Growth Factor Receptor

Truncated nerve growth factor receptor may serve as a marker of peripheral nerve injury and regeneration (Hruska et al., 1993), as truncated nerve growth factor receptor/creatinine ratios are increased in male and female patients with diabetic peripheral neuropathy with either type 1 or type 2 diabetes. These levels are not affected by the presence of proteinuria.

Symptoms Assessment

A large number of patients with diabetes report pain and paresthesias attributable to diabetic neuropathy. The reason for the appearance and severity of this pain is poorly understood. Britland et al. (1990) proposed that unequal rates of fiber regeneration may underlie differences in the extent of myelinated fiber loss between painful and painless diabetic polyneuropathy. However, they assert that myelinated and unmyelinated fiber degeneration and regeneration are probably not the cause of neuropathic pain in diabetic polyneuropathy *per se*, but that axonal atrophy may be involved in neuropathic pain generation. Given the prevalence of pain symptoms reported in patients with diabetes, it is important to accurately assess the nature, severity, and frequency of pain symptoms in controlled trials.

Total Symptom Score (TSS; Ziegler et al., 1995)

The TSS considers the intensity and frequency of four symptoms: pain, burning, paresthesias, and numbness. Scores from 0 (no symptoms) to 14.64 (all symptoms) are recorded. An abnormality is defined as a TSS greater than 0. An improvement in the TSS of approximately 30% (or at least 2 points in patients with up to 4 points at study entry) from baseline has been defined as a clinically meaningful difference. This scale has been shown to have some utility in the assessment of response to therapeutic agents in controlled trials. For example, Ziegler & Gries (1997) reported that TSS (in the feet) decreased from baseline to Day 19 with alpha-lipoic acid treatment versus placebo in patients with diabetic peripheral neuropathy.

McGill Pain Questionnaire (MPQ; Melzak, 1975)

The MPQ is designed to provide quantitative measures of clinical pain that can be treated statistically. The scale consists of three major classes of word descriptors (sensory, affective, and evaluative) that are used by patients to specify subjective pain experience. The MPQ also contains an intensity scale and other items to determine the properties of pain experience. The three major measures that can be derived from the questionnaire include the pain rating index (based on two types of numerical values that can be assigned to each word descriptor), the number of words chosen as applicable to the pain, and the present pain intensity based on a scale from 1 (mild) to 5 (excruciating). The MPQ is considered to be a reliable and accurate instrument for the assessment of pain in controlled clinical studies in various indications such as arthritis, migraine, and post-herpetic neuralgia. The MPQ is often utilized as a metric for the inclusion of patients in a study, while actual changes in pain associated with treatment are often assessed by other techniques such as the Visual Analog Scale.

Visual Analogue Scale (VAS)

The VAS is a simple tool that permits patients to rate the severity of their pain by placing a hatch mark on a line that ranges from *no pain* at the far left to *extreme pain* at the far right. Patients are given a diary to take home with space for completing the VAS once daily. Each evening, the patient completes the VAS, assessing the overall pain for that day. The diary can also contain a rescue medication section that documents the date and time of rescue medication administration with space for completing the VAS immediately prior to such administration. The VAS has been widely used in clinical trials across many different indications. For example, Ertas et al. (1998) reported that pain as measured by the VAS every week from Day 0 to Day 28 was helpful in discriminating patients who responded to levodopa for the control of painful diabetic neuropathy. In another study, patients who reported burning or formication on the MPQ experienced a significant reduction in pain associated with diabetic neuropathy as seen in the VAS after 5 weeks of treatment with mexiletine compared to placebo (Jarvis et al., 1998).

Neuropathic Pain Scale (NPS; Galer & Jensen, 1997)

The NPS is the first scale designed specifically to assess neuropathic pain. This scale consists of 10 items that are completed by the patient, and assesses various qualities of pain such as intensity (deep and surface), sensitivity, and unpleasantness, as well as a description of the time quality of pain. This test has been shown to have adequate discriminant and predictive validity in diabetic neuropathy, peripheral nerve injury, post-herpetic neuralgia, and complex regional pain syndrome. More importantly, this scale has been shown to be sensitive to treatments known to impact neuropathic pain, such as lidocaine and phentolamine, suggesting its utility in controlled clinical trials.

Strategies in Defining an Adequate Patient Population

Given the heterogeneity inherent in the expression of diabetic complications and the instability of this disorder, attempting to define a stable group of patients who may be suitable to assess therapeutic benefits in a controlled clinical trial is often a difficult task. This section is designed to provide some useful guidelines on the selection of appropriate patients for inclusion in such studies.

The first step in the identification of patients is to operationalize the notion of diabetic stability. Often this is defined as an HbA_{1c} concentration of 7.1–11.0% (inclusive), regardless of medication received. The range of permissible HbA_{1c} concentrations is often a subject of debate, but can be selected on the basis of published reports by researchers such as Adler et al., (1997), who identified poor glycemic control as a risk factor for both prevalent and incident neuropathy. Each percentage increase in baseline HbA_{1c} was associated with an approximate 15% increase in risk of neuropathy at follow-up examination. In addition, patients should be required to demonstrate symptomatic diabetic peripheral sensorimotor polyneuropathy at baseline (i.e., stage II Dyck criteria) using guidelines established by the San Antonio Criteria for Diabetic Neuropathy, which recommends at least one measure from each of the following categories to define and classify diabetic neuropathy: clinical symptoms, clinical examination, electrodiagnostic studies, quantitative sensory testing, and autonomic function testing. The investigation of stage II patients in clinical trials allows for a significant change in the dependant variables in either direction. Thus, there is a less likely chance of the dependent measure being confounded by the ceiling or floor effect often seen in very ill or newly ill patients.

Ideally, candidates for randomization should include those patients with established diabetes and a slowly progressive, symmetrical sensory/motor polyneuropathy. A baseline range of 30–45 m/s appears to be a good inclusion criterion for the peroneal motor nerve conduction velocity (PER-MNCV). This criterion is supported by both clinical and methodological considerations suggesting that: a) the majority of diabetic patients with

MNCV abnormalities and sural nerve pathology may be included within this range (Dyck et al., 1985); b) few patients with PER-MNCV abnormalities outside of this range have demonstrable sural nerve pathology; and c) a restriction in the sample for evaluation may have a favorable impact on the standard deviation of the measure. Patients with diabetic proximal motor neuropathy (e.g., diabetic amyotrophy) and patients whose neuropathy is predominantly characterized by a pronounced autonomic disturbance should be excluded, as should patients with focal and multi-focal neuropathies (cranial, trunk, limb, and asymmetric lower limb motor neuropathy).

Candidate patients should have a diagnosis of either type 1 or type 2 diabetes as defined by the National Diabetes Data Group, and have stable diabetes mellitus. As noted above, this may be operationalized as an HbA_{1c} level between 7.1 and 11.0% (inclusive). The presence of type 1 diabetes should also be documented by abnormal C peptide levels (≤ 0.2 ng/ml) at baseline. Candidate patients should exhibit one of the two abnormalities of PER-MNCV. For example, patients must have no more than moderate symmetrical sensory polyneuropathy as characterized by their ability to walk on heels, bilateral sural nerve amplitudes above detection threshold, or bilateral vibratory thresholds in the great toe >4.0 μm and <40μm (inclusive).

Candidate patients should not have moderate-to-severe uncontrolled hypertension (diastolic blood pressure ≥ 105 mmHg). Candidate patients should not have any other causes of peripheral neuropathy (e.g., inflammatory/demyelinating, infectious granulomatous, endocrine (hypothyroidism, acromegaly), neuropathy secondary to alcoholism or nutritional metabolic disturbance, or neuropathies which are a reflection of ischemic injury, paraproteinemias, malignancy, or toxic agents. Finally, candidate patients should not have isolated asymmetrical mononeuropathy of trunk or limb, asymmetric lower limb motor neuropathy, cranial neuropathy, or clinically important evidence of autonomic neuropathy secondary to diabetes (e.g., clinical evidence of gastrointestinal autonomic neuropathy that may alter drug absorption).

Analytic Strategies in Diabetic Neuropathy

In controlled studies designed to assess the effects of various therapeutic agents on diabetic neuropathy, the primary efficacy objective is usually to demonstrate a statistically significant difference between therapeutic agents and placebo. As such, the primary statistical analysis typically involves some electrophysiological index, such as PER-MNCV, as an estimate of neuropathic severity over time. Any changes from baseline to endpoint (last patient observed time) can be then be analyzed using an identified intent-to-treat population. An analysis of covariance (ANCOVA) model with the baseline PER-MNCV, treatment, and site as factors can be used to accomplish this. Examples of other common statistical covariates include age, duration of illness, and various measures of glycemic control. When there is a concern that there may be a bias introduced by chance covariate imbalance, a W statistic that measures change from baseline can be utilized. However, this test is less powerful than ANCOVA (Donahue, 1997).

Another example of a specific efficacy variable that might be evaluated in proposed clinical trials involves the specific slope corresponding to the average rate of disease progression with respect to time for each patient. The slope can be estimated by fitting a simple linear regression model of MNCV versus time to all available therapy values for that patient.

Model adequacy can be assessed, and if sufficient, descriptive summaries can also be provided for the derived slope overall and with respect to treatment group. The analysis for this endpoint can include an ANCOVA of the patient's specific slopes, with treatment groups and study centers as factors, and with the baseline conduction velocity as a covariate. Exploratory analyses can include model development procedures considering at least age, gender, disease duration, and various clinical scale scores (such as the NSS, NDS and TSS) at baseline as possible contributory factors. The NDS, NSS, and TSS can also be analyzed individually as change scores, using analytical approaches as defined above.

An integrated summary statistic (dependent variable) can also be developed for each patient utilizing a combination of any number of the above dependent measures. For example, the rank scores of the PER-MNCV, NDS, NSS, and SIP total score are all available possible endpoints, and therefore can be aggregated to form an integrated measure. Each efficacy variable can be standardized through ranking procedures. Subsequently, treatment and dose effects can be evaluated across both the primary and secondary hypotheses, using standard analytic procedures.

Another technique that takes into account multiple dependent measures is the "global" test. This test was utilized in the t-PA Stroke Trial where clinician participants advocated categorizing outcomes as favorable/unfavorable, and agreed that a global test was appropriate for ischemic stroke when no single outcome is accepted (Tilley et al., 1996). Finally, it is possible to construct composite test scores, as seen in the following chapter regarding diabetes-related cognitive dysfunction. Briefly, this method involves the use of normative data to create Z transformed values for each dependent measure. These transformed scores can then be appropriately weighed in composite scales based on current research and theory regarding diabetic neuropathy. Separate composite scales can be made for pain measures, electrophysiological measures, and standard clinical measures. It is also possible to construct such composite scores based on statistical findings from raw or transformed data derived from techniques such as factor analysis. Composite scales can then be constructed on the basis of their factor loadings. These composite scales suggested by the factor loadings can then be further refined based on the internal consistency of each summary scale as assessed through coefficient alphas or inter-item covariance statistical procedures.

The variability of individual markers of diabetic neuropathy has resulted in the increased use and acceptance of composite test scores in recent years. Another approach to the use of composite test scores proposed by Dyck et al. (1997) has met with considerable success in both the diagnosis of diabetic neuropathy and in the accurate assessment of change over time and treatment conditions. This approach utilizes a percentile cutoff score based on a combination of several measures. Specifically, this group reported that a composite score consisting of the Neuropathy Impairment Score of the lower limbs plus seven additional tests provided a better minimal criteria of diabetic neuropathy than clinical judgment or any previously published minimal criteria based on one or two impairments obtained from multiple measures. This composite score, referred to as the NSS(LL)+7, was found to be useful in detecting worsening of patients with diabetes and diabetic polyneuropathy in a population-based study. The rate of decline (0.34 points for diabetic patients and 0.85 points for patients with diabetic polyneuropathy) over one year suggests that a controlled clinical trial would have to last for a period of three years in order to observe a deterioration in an untreated control group of 2 NIS points, a change considered to be clinically meaningful by the Peripheral Nerve Society. It is assumed that most anti-neuropathic therapies are unlikely to improve nerve function but instead can only halt or slow progression of the disease. For such therapies, a clinically meaningful treatment effect cannot be detected by this composite approach until three years' deterioration is accrued in the untreated group. The authors also determined that at least 70 patients under 65 years of age will be required in each arm of the trial to achieve adequate statistical power.

Regulatory Perspective

Following the disappointing results from trials of various aldose reductase inhibitors for the treatment of diabetic neuropathy, the FDA has attempted to facilitate the development of such treatments by entertaining discussion on any outcome approach that might reasonably predict long-term clinical benefit. An example is provided by the morphometric evaluation of biopsied nerve tissue. It was proposed that a standardized characterization of various features of nerve regeneration and density would provide an early, sensitive, and accurate indication of therapeutic benefit. The Agency was willing to accept these outcomes as the basis for providing one of the two pivotal trials necessary for approval of an indication for neuropathy. Several trials were conducted with nerve morphometry as the primary outcome. Unfortunately, the variability of the parameters used for this evaluation and other technical problems undermined the biostatistical power of these trials. Given these shortcomings and the invasiveness of this approach, peripheral nerve morphometry can no longer be considered a viable means of assessing efficacy.

However, one important side benefit of developing the nerve biopsy approach is that drug penetration, and in the case of aldose reductase inhibitors, enzyme inhibition, can be measured at the target tissue. This use of nerve biopsy has proved to be a crucial step in verifying that dose regimens of anti-neuropathic therapies provide adequate drug exposure at the nerve. For this purpose, far fewer patients are needed. It is debatable, however, whether nerve biopsy is ethically acceptable in patients or in normal subjects since the biopsy results in permanent sensory loss, albeit very small and localized, in the distribution of the sampled nerve.

Two thorny issues now face evaluators of anti-neuropathy therapies. The first is the level of glycemic control that should be required in patients participating in these trials. Some Agency reviewers have said that not only should reasonable glycemic control be aimed for but that good glycemic control should be achieved in these trials. On the one hand, it is probably true that the conditions of a clinical trial can achieve what cannot or will not be achieved in the real world. On the other hand, clinical trials should attempt to simulate, within ethical bounds, the conditions that exist in real world practice. An anti-neuropathy therapy trial, which mandates improved glycemic control, is in effect testing two hypotheses at the same time. One of these interventions, i.e., improved glycemic control, is not likely to be sustained once the trial is over. The Agency is better advised to ask that good standards of glycemic care be incorporated in neuropathy trials, but that efforts not be required that exceed what is achievable in everyday practice.

The other issue faced by the Agency is caused by the composite approach for assessing efficacy. Reporting the results of multiple neurophysiologic and symptomatic outcomes with a single summary statistic is the most appropriate means of expressing these outcomes when it is unknown *a priori* which single or few outcomes are the most robust and/or predictive measures of a clinical benefit. The composite approach of Dyck et al. discussed above is based on longitudinal epidemiologic data and thereby has achieved a certain level of validation. The drawback here is that the summary statistic provided by this and other composite approaches is abstract and not readily understood by the clinician. The approach of Dyck et al. has the attractive feature of a stated magnitude of effect that is considered by the authors to be clinically meaningful. This recommendation makes it easy for regulators who want to have a bright line for defining efficacy, but will be a source of consternation for developers with treatment effects that fall short of the line.

A final regulatory distinction should be made between an indication for improvement of neuropathic pain and an indication for slowing the progression of diabetic neuropathy. The effectiveness of therapies that are, in effect, specialized analgesics for treatment of neuropathic pain can be evaluated in relatively short trials comparable to trials with which other analgesic therapies are evaluated. The only proviso that has been articulated by FDA's Metabolic and Endocrine division in the case of palliative therapies for diabetic neuropathic pain is that an adequate safety examination reveals no adverse effect on nerve function. The monitoring of nerve conduction velocity or composite measures of nerve function over a 12-month period would probably suffice to provide this assurance.

DIABETIC NEPHROPATHY

Diabetic nephropathy is the third major microvascular complication and the most important in terms of economic impact. Diabetic nephropathy is the most common cause of end-stage renal disease (ESRD) and dialysis dependency in the industrialized world. The importance of this disorder and the rapidly expanding knowledge about its pathophysiology warrant a separate chapter or even an entire book. These reasons along with the fact that a major trial of an anti-nephropathy therapy is about to be reported render a comprehensive discussion of this complication beyond the reach of this book. Instead, some of the main points about developing therapies for diabetic nephropathy will be covered only briefly here with a commitment to provide a full treatment of the subject in the near future.

Captopril (Capoten,™ Bristol-Myers Squibb Co.), an angiotensin-converting enzyme inhibitor (ACE inhibitor) originally approved for the treatment of hypertension, is the only therapy to be approved by the FDA for a diabetic complication. The approval of the indication for diabetic nephropathy was based on captopril's beneficial effects on renal function and progression to ESRD. The therapy is indicated in patients with 24-hour urinary protein excretion exceeding 500 mg. ACE inhibitor therapy has become standard therapy for patients with proteinuria of any degree even though its benefit on slowing progression to renal failure for patients with protein excretion below 500 mg has not been established. Two trials have demonstrated a benefit of captopril on progression to overt proteinuria in patients with 20-200 μg/min. ACE inhibitor therapy has become an attractive choice for treating hypertension uncomplicated by proteinuria in patients with diabetes largely because of the anticipation that this therapy will forestall the development of renal dysfunction.

Captopril's efficacy is substantial, but provides only about half that needed. Complementary therapeutic approaches should be pursued to fully avert the development of nephropathy. Because captopril has become a standard therapy, the development of new therapies will be more challenging. The therapeutic window for subsequent treatments is considerably smaller since no nephropathy trial can be ethically conducted without ACE inhibitor therapy. For example, captopril therapy itself might have fallen short of producing statistically significant treatment effects in the same trials on which approval was based if a comparably effective background therapy had been available.

The other major obstacle for development of additional therapies aimed at preventing nephropathy is the strong secular trend in risk factor reduction for this complication. Improved glycemic and blood lipid control, decreased smoking, earlier detection and treatment of microalbuminuria all serve to lower the rate of progression to renal dysfunction and ESRD. Thus, the absolute treatment effect being pursued in the development of new therapies continues to shrink. It should be recognized, however, that a substantial number of patients will progress to disabling nephropathy despite captopril therapy. Captopril itself is not risk free. This therapy is recognized to cause anaphylactic-like reactions, angioedema, neutropenia/agranulocytosis, and increased proteinuria with occasional nephrotic syndrome.

Regulatory authorities should therefore take these considerations into account in adjusting the requirements for therapies aimed at prevention and treatment of diabetic nephropathy. One possible approach is the use of well-accepted surrogate outcomes. The leading candidate for this role is proteinuria. In the original captopril trial, protein excretion was reduced by 30% in the first 3 months of captopril therapy and this reduction was maintained for the rest of the trial. A large body of evidence now supports the view that excreted protein itself is a tubular toxin. Proteinuria is now regarded by some experts as not only a reflection of dysfunction for all glomerulopathies, but as a common etiologic pathway on which all these diseases converge (Cartran et al., 1994). Reduction of protein excretion regardless of cause could thereby be justified as a therapeutic objective. By extension, protein excretion could be accepted as a reasonable surrogate if not an outright clinical outcome on which a nephropathy indication could be based.

Those with a more conservative perspective will still insist that the same kind of outcomes like ESRD and mortality found to be improved in the captopril trial also be asked of developers of new therapies. Though some evaluators within FDA may hold this view, senior FDA officials have informally indicated willingness to accept clinically meaningful treatment effects on renal function as sufficient for justifying approval. Because of the accumulation of important, unsettled issues for developing nephropathy therapies, the FDA should hold an advisory committee hearing to provide resolution and clarity in this therapeutic area.

CONCLUSIONS

Complications related to diabetes in the form of diabetic retinopathy, neuropathy, and nephropathy account for a significant proportion of associated morbidity and mortality in this disease. Therefore, it is essential that novel therapeutic agents be developed and rigorously tested with the hope of targeting some of the symptoms associated with these complications. The successful study of such agents can be aided through the use of reliable and valid measures of diabetic microvascular complications in randomized, double-blind, placebo-controlled clinical trials. Some of the more useful and accepted assessment procedures used to assess the presence of diabetic retinopathy, neuropathy, and nephropathy (as well as changes related to treatment) have been provided above. Additionally, many of these measures have been used to detect some degree of efficacy in prior experimental studies. The single best technique that allows for the accurate detection of diabetic retinopathy, as well as quantification of changes in retinopathic status over time (or treatment) is seven-standard field fundus photography. This technique is generally accepted as the gold standard in assessment of diabetic retinopathy and has shown adequate sensitivity in numerous controlled clinical trials. In contrast, there is no comparable standard for the assessment of diabetic neuropathy.

Electrophysiological measures such as PER-MNCV remain the preferred primary measure in traditional nerve conduction studies, as they are a principal objective measure of functional integrity in diabetic sensorimotor neuropathy. Comprehensive clinical neurological evaluations such as the NDS and the NSS can also help to characterize changes in the neuropathic condition at baseline and throughout treatment. Specialized scales to assess pain and QOL measures may also serve as useful markers of disease progression and treatment response. Finally, a composite metric consisting of multiple dependent measures, such as that seen in the integrated summary statistic, has shown some utility in the evaluation of treatment response. Protein excretion has emerged as the leading candidate for therapeutic outcome in the assessment of diabetic nephropathy, although a clarification of regulatory expectations is necessary. The application and utility of these various assessment techniques depends largely upon the nature and scope of the clinical trial being conducted, as well as the type of patients being studied. However, regardless of the type of trial being initiated or patient type, it is necessary to address issues surrounding the heterogeneity of symptom expression, and the disease instability inherent in diabetic retinopathy, neuropathy, and nephropathy. Finally, important moderator variables and risk factors known to affect the prevalence and severity of these diabetic complications should be carefully considered in the design of controlled clinical trials.

References

Adler AI, Boyko EJ, Ahroni JH, Stensel V, Forsberg RC, Smith DG. Risk factors for diabetic peripheral sensory neuropathy: results of the Seattle Prospective Disease Foot Study. *Diabetes Care* 1997; **20**: 1162.

Aldington SJ, Kohner EM, Meuer S, Klein R, Sjolie AK. Methodology for retinal photography and assessment of diabetic retinopathy: The EURODIAB IDDM complications study. *Diabetologia* 1995; **38**(4): 437–44.

Allen L. Ocular fundus photography. *Am J Ophthalmol* 1964; **57**: 13–28.

Arend O, Remky A, Evans D, Stuber R, Harris A. Contrast sensitivity loss is coupled with dropout in patients with diabetes. *Invest Ophthalmol Vis Sci* 1997; **38**(9): 1819–24.

Bergner M, Bobbit RA, Carter WB, Gilson BS. The sickness impact profile: development and final revision of a health status measure. *Med Care* 1981; **19**: 787–805.

Britland ST, Young RJ, Sharma AK, Clarke BF. Association of painful and painless diabetic polyneuropathy with different patterns of nerve fiber degeneration and regeneration. *Diabetes* 1990; **39**(8): 898–908.

Cartran DC, Greenwood C, Ritchie S. Long-term benefit of angiotensin-converting enzyme inhibitor therapy in patients with severe immunoglobulin A nephropathy: a comparison to patients receiving treatment with other antihypertensive agents and to patients receiving no therapy. *Am J Kidney Dis* 1994; **23**: 247–54.

Cunha-Vaz J. Lowering the risk of visual impairment and blindness. *Diabet Med* 1998; **15**(Suppl 4): S47–50.

Danne T, Kordonouri O, Enders I, Hovener G, Weber B. Factors modifying the effect of hyperglycemia on the development of retinopathy in adolescents with diabetes. Results of the Berlin Retinopathy Study. *Horm Res* 1998; **50**(Suppl)1: 28–32.

Davis MD. Worsening of diabetic retinopathy after improvement of glycemic control. *Arch Ophthalmol* 1998; **116**(7): 931–932.

DCCT Research Group. The effect of intensive treatment of diabetes on the development and progression of long-term complications in insulin-dependent diabetes mellitus. *N Engl J Med* 1993; **329**: 977–987.

Deschenes MC, Coupland SG, Ross SA, Fick GH. Early macular dysfunction detected by focal electroretinographic recording in non-insulin-dependent diabetics without retinopathy. *Doc Ophthalmol* 1997–98; **94**(3): 223–37.

The Diabetic Retinopathy Study Research Group. Preliminary report on effects of photocoagulation therapy. *Am J Ophthalmol* 1976; **81**: 1.

The Diabetic Retinopathy Study Research Group. Photocoagulation treatment of proliferative diabetic retinopathy: The second report of diabetic retinopathy study findings. *Ophthalmology* 1978; **85**: 82.

Donahue RM. A summary statistic for measuring change from baseline. *J Biopharm Stat* 1997; **7**(2): 287–299.

Dyck PJ. Detection, characterization, and staging of polyneuropathy assessed in diabetics. *Muscle & Nerve* 1988; **11**: 21–32.

Dyck PJ, Davies JL, Litchy WJ, O'Brien. Longitudinal assessment of diabetic polyneuropathy using a composite score in the Rochester Diabetic Neuropathy Study cohort. *Neurology* 1997; **49**(1): 229–39.

Dyck PJ, Karnes JL, Daube J, O'Brien P, Service FJ. Clinical and neuropathological criteria for the diagnosis and staging of diabetic polyneuropathy. *Brain* 1985; **108**: 861–880.

Dyck PJ, Kratz KM, Lehman KA, Karnes JL, Melton LJ 3rd, O'Brien PC, Litchy WJ, Windebank AJ, Smith BE, Low PA, et al. The Rochester Diabetic Neuropathy Study: design, criteria for types of neuropathy, selection bias, and reproducibility of neuropathic tests. *Neurology* 1991; **41**: 799–807.

Dyck PJ, Sherman WR, Hallacher LM, Service FJ, O'Brien PC, Grina LA, Palumbo PJ. Swanson CJ. Human diabetic endoneurial sorbitol, fructose, and myo-inositol related to sural nerve morphometry. *Ann Neurol* 1980; **8**: 590–596.

Dyck PJ, Zimmerman IR, O'Brien PC, Ness A, Caskey PE, Karnes J, Bushek W. Introduction of automated systems to evaluate touch-pressure, vibration and thermal cutaneous sensation in man. *Ann Neurol* 1978; **4**: 502–510.

Early Treatment Diabetic Retinopathy Study: Report Number 4. Photocoagulatioin for diabetic macular edema. *Int Ophthalmol Clin* 1987; **27**: 265–272.

Ertas M, Sagduyu A, Arac N, Uludag B, Ertekin C. Use of levodopa to relieve pain from painful symmetrical diabetic polyneuropathy. *Pain* 1998; **75**(2–3): 257–9.

Ewing FM, Deary IJ, Strachan MW, Frier BM. Seeing beyond retinopathy in diabetes: electrophysiological and psychophysical abnormalities and alterations in vision. *Endocr Rev* 1998 Aug; **19**(4): 462–76.

Fujio N, Yoshida A, Ogasawara H, Feke GT, McMeel JW. The new laser Doppler velocimetry for the measurement of retinal circulation and its clinical application. *Hokkaido Igaku Zasshi* 1996; **71**(6): 757–69.

Galer BS, Jensen MP. Development and preliminary validation of a pain measure specific to neuropathic pain: The Neuropathic Pain Scale. *Neurology* 1997; 48: 332–338.

Gilbert RE; Tsalamandris C; Allen TJ; Colville D; Jerums G. Early nephropathy predicts vision-threatening retinal disease in patients with type I diabetes mellitus. *J Am Soc Nephrol* 1998; **9**(1): 85–89.

Gregersen G. Diabetic neuropathy: influence of age, sex, metabolic control and duration of diabetes on motor conduction velocity. *Neurology* 1967; **17**: 972–980.

Guy RJC, Clark CA, Malcolm PN, Watkins PJ. Evaluation of thermal and vibration sensation in diabetic neuropathy. *Diabetologia* 1985; **28**: 131–137.

Hruska RE, Chertack MM, Kravis, D. Elevation of nerve growth factor receptor-truncated in the urine of patients with diabetic neuropathy. *Ann NY Acad Sci* 1993; **679**: 349–351.

Ishiko S, Yoshida A, Mori F, Abiko T, Kitaya N, Konno S, Kato Y. Corneal and lens autofluorescence in young insulin-dependent diabetic patients. *Ophthalm* 1998; **212**(5): 301–5.

Jarvis B, Coukell AJ. Mexiletine. A review of its therapeutic use in painful diabetic neuropathy. *Drugs* 1998; **56**(4): 691–707.

Jeddi A, Ben Osman N, Daghfous F, Kaoueche M, Baccar M, Gaigi S, Ayed S. Methods for screening and surveillance of diabetic retinopathy. *J Fr Ophtalmol* 1994; **17**(12): 769–73.

Kennedy WR, Wendelschafer-Crabb. Quantification of nerve in skin biopsies for control in diabetic subjects. *Soc Neurosci Abs* 1994; 70.

Klein R, Klein BEK. Diabetic eye disease. *Lancet* 1997; **350**: 197–204.

McNair DM, Lorr M, Droppleman LF. *Manual for the Profile of Mood States.* San Diego:

Educational & Industrial Testing Service, 1971.

Melzak R. The McGill pain questionnaire: major properties and scoring methods. *Pain* 1975; **1**:277–299.

Mendvil A, Cuartero V. Ocular blood flow velocities in patients with proliferative diabetic retinopathy after scatter photocoagulation. Two years of follow-up. *Retina* 1996; 16(3): 222–227.

Merbis MA, Snoek FJ, Kanc K, Heine RJ. Hypoglycaemia induces emotional disruption. *Patient Educ Couns* 1996; **29**(1): 117–122.

Negrin P, Zara G. Conduction studies as prognostic parameters in the natural history of diabetic neuropathy: a long-term follow-up of 114 patients. *Electromyogr Clin Neurophysiol* 1995; **35**(6):341–50.

Pfeiffer MA, Peterson H, Dyck PJ, Thomas PK, Asbury AK, Winegard AI, Porte D Jr. (eds). Cardiovascular autonomic neuropathy. In: *Diabetic Neuropathy*. Philadelphia: WB Saunders, 1987, pp. 122-133.

Rajala U, Laakso M, Qiao Q, Keinanen-Kiukaanniemi S. Prevalence of retinopathy in people with diabetes, impaired glucose tolerance, and normal glucose tolerance. *Diabetes Care* 1998; **21**(10): 1664–1669.

Rose M, Burkert U, Scholler G, Schirop T, Danzer G, Klapp BF. Determinants of the quality of life of patients with diabetes under intensified insulin therapy. *Diabetes Care* 1998; **21**(11): 1876–85.

Shaw JE, Gokal R, Hollis S, Boulton AJ. Does peripheral neuropathy invariably accompany nephropathy in type 1 diabetes mellitus? *Diabetes Res Clin Pract* 1998; **39**(1): 55–61.

Silvers D, Kipnes M, Broadstone V, Patterson D, Quigley EM, McCallum R, Leidy NK, Farup C, Liu Y, Joslyn A. Domperidone in the management of symptoms of diabetic gastroparesis: efficacy, tolerability, and quality-of-life outcome sin a multicenter controlled trial. DOM-USA-5 Study Group. *Clin Ther* 1998; **20**(3): 438–453.

The Sorbinil Retinopathy Trial Research Group. A randomized trial of sorbinil, an aldose reductase inhibitor in diabetic retinopathy. *Arch Ophthalmol* 1990; **108**:1234–1244.

Tilley BC, Marler J, Geller NL, Lu M, Legler J, Brott T, Lyden P, Grotta J. Use of a global test for multiple outcomes in stroke trials with application to the National Institute of Neurological Disorders and Stroke t-PA Stroke Trial. *Stroke* 1996; **27**(11): 2136–2142.

Yu T, Mitchell P, Berry G, Li W, Wang JJ. Retinopathy in older persons without diabetes and its relationship to hypertension. *Arch Ophthalmol* 1998; **116**(1): 83–89.

Vijan S, Hofer TP, Hayward RA. Estimated benefits of glycemic control on microvascular complications in type 2 diabetes. *Ann Intern Med* 1997; **127**(9): 788–795.

Weinberger M, Kirkman MS, Samsa GP, Cowper PA, Shortliffe E, Simel DL, Feussner JR. The relationship between glycemic control and health-related quality of life in patients with non-insulin-dependent diabetes mellitus. *Med Care* 1994; **32**(123): 1173–1181.

Ziegler D, Hanefeld M, Ruhnau KJ, Meissner HP, Lobisch M, Schutte K, Gries FA. Treatment of symptomatic diabetic peripheral neuropathy with the anti-oxidant α-lipoic acid: a 3-week multicentre randomized controlled trial (ALADIN study). *Diabetologia* 1995; **38**: 1425-1433.

Ziegler D, Gries FA. Alpha-lipoic acid in the treatment of diabetic peripheral and cardiac autonomic neuropathy. *Diabetes* 1997; **46**(Suppl 2): S62-6.

11

METHODOLOGICAL CONSIDERATIONS: DIABETES-RELATED COGNITIVE DYSFUNCTION

Although it has long been recognized that severe cases of diabetes can result in central nervous system (CNS) disturbances through the various mechanisms involved in cerebrovascular accidents, more recent evidence has suggested that even mild forms of diabetes can interfere with CNS functioning in the absence of overt cerebrovascular accidents or repeated hypoglycemic reactions (Mooradian, 1997). This is not surprising, considering that the nervous system functions as a unit, and that microvascular changes in diabetes have long been shown to result in the disruption of the local circulation to various organ systems including the peripheral nervous system and retina. Moreover, post-mortem analyses have suggested that chronic and poorly-controlled diabetes is associated with degenerative changes in the brain. The association between diabetes and CNS dysfunction has been observed in patients with type 1 and type 2 diabetes, as well as in animal models of experimentally-induced diabetes. In humans, this dysfunction often manifests itself in the form of mild cognitive impairment. However, the extent and nature of diabetes-related cognitive impairment remains largely unknown. This is largely due to poorly-controlled and underpowered investigations of experimentally-manipulated glycemic control, and a paucity of controlled clinical trials that have utilized measures of cognitive dysfunction when assessing therapeutic efficacy. Thus, the notion of central impairment in diabetes, often labeled as "central neuropathy" or "diabetic encephalopathy," has not gained wide recognition or acceptance.

The potential causes of CNS dysfunction in diabetes can be classified broadly into vascular causes (including changes in the blood-brain barrier) and metabolic changes (Mooradian, 1997). The latter includes objective manifestations such as repeated hypoglycemic episodes, hyperglycemia, hyperosmolality, acidosis, ketosis, and various neuroendocrine and neurochemical changes. There are also other potential contributory causes of CNS dysfunction in diabetes that include the presence of complicating features such as hypertension, uremia, and peripheral and autonomic neuropathy. It is more likely that CNS dysfunction is the end product of a yet unknown set of complex interactions between metabolic abnormalities, diabetes-related complications, and more direct mechanisms of neural damage (e.g., those seen with NMDA or excitotoxins). One such theory by Messier (1996) postulates that the mechanisms involved in poor glycemic control somehow potentiate the neuronal death produced by other pathological processes, such as amyloid deposition in Alzheimer's disease.

A strong relationship between diabetes and Alzheimer's disease has been postulated by several researchers over the past decade. For example, L'Hommedieu and Podraza (1989), in their bibliography of cognitive studies in diabetes, proposed that diabetes may represent a form of "accelerated aging." Additionally, as part of the Rotterdam study, Ott et al. (1996) suggested a positive association between diabetes and dementia (odds ratio 1.3). The relationship was strongest between diabetes and vascular dementia, but an association was also observed with Alzheimer's disease. These associations were independent of age, education, and risk factors such as smoking, body mass index, atherosclerosis, and hypertension.

An association between Alzheimer's disease and diabetes was also noted by Hershey et al. (1997), who proposed that the cerebral structures implicated in Alzheimer's disease and memory function are also more prone to the effects of hypoglycemia. Further, they hypothesized that the deleterious effect of hypoglycemia on medial temporal structures such as the hippocampus helps to explain the finding that while declarative memory function is impaired in type 1 diabetic patients, nondeclarative memory is relatively spared. Fushimi et al. (1996) proposed a more direct mechanism of cerebral damage in diabetes by examining the relationship between the presence of lacunae on magnetic resonance imaging (MRI) and multiple risk factors for type 2 diabetes such as age, hypertension, and hyperlipidemia in asymptomatic type 2 diabetic patients and healthy controls. A 42% incidence of lacunae was revealed in the diabetic patients, with older patients having the highest incidence. Additionally, the presence of lacunae was associated with global measures of intellectual impairment.

In addition to the above studies, there is a growing body of evidence from case studies, epidemiological evaluations, quasi-experimental investigations, controlled clinical trials, and studies of experimentally-induced changes in glycemic control which indicates that type 1 and type 2 diabetes are associated with cerebral dysfunction manifested primarily by mild cognitive impairment. Importantly, it has also been established that this impairment may be amenable to treatment. However, this mild level of cognitive dysfunction often goes undetected upon routine clinical evaluation and may only be apparent under conditions of heightened cognitive demands which are achieved with standardized evaluations of highly specialized and sensitive neuropsychological assessment procedures.

STUDIES OF EXPERIMENTALLY-INDUCED CHANGES IN GLYCEMIC CONTROL

One of the first attempts to utilize experimental manipulations of glycemic control came from Hoffman et al. (1989), who examined 18 type 1 diabetic patients under conditions of hypoglycemia, normoglycemia, and hyperglycemia. Glycemic conditions were maintained by an insulin/glucose infusion system and were counterbalanced for each subject in a single-blind, repeated-measures design. These researchers reported that performance on measures of visual tracking, visuomotor speed, concentration, and mental flexibility (Trail Making B) were impaired in hypoglycemic compared to normoglycemic conditions. This specific impairment on visual and executive measures suggests a pattern of right hemisphere and frontal system dysfunction in type 1 diabetic patients that has been reproduced many times.

As many neuropsychological tests have a motor component, it is important to attempt to decompose the nature of the neuropsychological impairment observed upon assessment. Specifically, one must assess whether changes in neuropsychological function during experimentally-induced hypoglycemia are due primarily to motor difficulties, or are more attributable to deficits in higher cognitive functioning. One study that helped to address this issue was conducted by Cox et al. (1993), who assessed diabetic patients at various levels of euglycemia and hypoglycemia on measures of pure motor functioning and pure cognitive functioning. They reported that diabetic patients exhibited impairment at blood glucose nadir (2.6 mmol/L), and concluded that cognitive tasks were more sensitive to these effects than motor tasks. This finding refutes prior notions that neuropsychological impairment is primarily due to motor difficulties (secondary to peripheral neuropathy) and confirms the importance of using measures with high cognitive demands when attempting to uncover diabetes-related cognitive difficulties.

Research by Draelos et al., (1995) supported the role of higher cognitive dysfunction in diabetic patients by demonstrating deficits in all areas of cognitive function during experimentally-induced hypoglycemia that were apparent irrespective of prior glycemic control. Interestingly, no deficits were seen during episodes of hyperglycemia. Specifically, the cognitive domains most affected during hypoglycemia included measures of associative learning, attention, and mental flexibility. Finally, these researchers reported that females were less cognitively impaired at the lowest level of hypoglycemia (2.2 mmol/L) than males, suggesting a gender-mediated effect on cognitive dysfunction in diabetes. It is possible that estrogen may somehow exert a protective effect against the hypoglycemia-mediated neural disruption. In addition to gender, there are many other important modifying variables and risk factors that must be taken into consideration in the examination of cognitive dysfunction in diabetes.

MODERATING VARIABLES IMPORTANT IN DIABETES-RELATED COGNITIVE DYSFUNCTION

In addition to experimentally-induced models of hypoglycemia, there have been numerous other reports suggesting a "central" impairment or encephalopathy in diabetes. These studies have demonstrated the importance of carefully examining various modifying, secondary, and potential independent variables in the study of diabetes-related cognitive dysfunction. These demographic, biomedical, and psychosocial risk factors have been shown to increase the risk of developing cognitive impairment in type 1 and type 2 diabetes. Some of the more salient variables include duration of illness, degree of metabolic control, history of severe hypoglycemic episodes, presence of hypoglycemic unawareness, type of treatment intervention (conventional versus intensive), gender, ethnicity, depression, and various diabetes-related complications (e.g., nephropathy, retinopathy, and peripheral and autonomic neuropathy). Further, there are numerous variables known to affect neuropsychological functioning that are disease irrelevant. These include age, gender, educational level, premorbid intellectual functioning, socioeconomic status, and various neurobehavioral risk factors such as alcohol use, head injury with loss of consciousness, and learning disorders. Given their suspected role in the genesis and maintenance of diabetes-related cognitive dysfunction, it is extremely important to quantify and attempt to experimentally control for these variables when designing a study to assess the effects of diabetes on cognitive function. This can be achieved through randomization procedures (provided sample sizes are large enough) or by building these variables into the study design through careful experimental manipulation including systematization, stratification, matching, conservative arrangement, or simply eliminating subjects with the variable altogether. When these steps are not possible or practical (as when using available samples), the variables should still be quantified, as the option of statistical covariance of these variables at the conclusion of the study may be warranted.

Duration of Illness

One of the most important variables mediating the relationship between diabetes and cognitive impairment is duration of illness. As seen in many chronic disorders, the duration of illness is an important factor that is often intrinsically tied to various measures of disease severity. Prescott et al. (1990) reported that the duration of illness in type 1 diabetes was inversely related to performance on memory measures, with more pronounced effects on the encoding of concrete rather than abstract material. However, this group reported that the degree of glycemic control in their patients was not related to performance, leading them to assert that the cognitive impairment associated with diabetes is more likely due to the impact of suffering a life-threatening disease than to organic damage *per se*. However, it is difficult to disentangle the effects of chronicity from the disease-specific effects of diabetes, based on the lack of correlation with glycemic control.

Other researchers, such as Croxson and Jagger (1995), reported that diabetes (as measured by glucose tolerance) was associated with a global measure of cognitive dysfunction (the Mini-Mental State Examination [MMSE]). These researchers reported that subjects with known diabetes were 3.3 times more likely than normal control subjects to have low MMSE scores (below 24); while newly-diagnosed diabetic patients were less likely to have MMSE scores below this cutoff. This cutoff is considered to be an accurate metric for identifying patients with significant cognitive impairment.

Finally, Ziegler et al. (1994) reported that the cerebral glucose consumption of [^{18}F]fluorodeoxyglucose (measured by positron emission tomography) was significantly reduced in chronic diabetic patients (who had symptoms of neuropathy) as compared to newly-diagnosed patients. Importantly, cerebral glucose metabolism was inversely correlated with the duration of diabetes and age (which is often confounded with duration of illness and age of onset).

Severe Hypoglycemic Episodes

The relationship between severe hypoglycemic episodes and cognitive dysfunction in type 1 diabetes has been investigated by many researchers. For example, Wredling et al. (1990) reported that patients with recurrent, severe hypoglycemic episodes scored lower than those with no history of severe hypoglycemia on tests of motor ability, short-term and associative memory, and visual spatial tasks assessing general problem-solving abilities. Additionally, these authors reported that patients with severe hypoglycemic episodes had a significantly higher frequency of perspective reversals, suggesting frontal lobe involvement that may represent a permanent neuropsychological impairment.

Langan et al. (1991) examined two groups of type 1 diabetic patients that were stratified on the basis of history of severe hypoglycemia (patients in one group had never experienced an episode while patients in the other group had experienced at least five episodes). The groups were balanced on measures of premorbid IQ, age, and duration of diabetes. These authors reported that patients with a history of at least five episodes of severe hypoglycemia had greater intellectual impairment and larger reaction time variances in comparison to patients with no history of severe hypoglycemia. Additionally, significant correlations were noted between the frequency of severe hypoglycemic episodes and the estimated magnitude of intellectual decline, performance IQ, and reaction time, with patients who had more episodes of hypoglycemia exhibiting poorer performance.

Similarly, Lincoln et al. (1996) reported a significant correlation between apparent decline in intellectual functioning (operationalized as a premorbid intellectual estimate minus actual IQ) and the frequency of major hypoglycemic events. However, they reported few differences in cognitive function between patients with or without a history of recurrent hypoglycemia, suggesting that dichotomizing patients based on the presence of this variable may have resulted in some loss of sensitivity in characterizing this relationship. Given the above studies, history of glycemic episodes appears to be an important risk factor for developing diabetes-related cognitive dysfunction, and therefore should be carefully considered when designing studies attempting to maximize effects between patient groups.

Hypoglycemic Unawareness

Hypoglycemic unawareness is a construct used to identify the conditions surrounding the lack of perceived knowledge of, or poor vigilance for, symptoms of glycemic changes, which include hunger, facial flushing, trembling, and sweating. This construct is important in that it may serve as a mediating variable in the relationship between hypoglycemia and cognitive dysfunction. For example, in an examination of the impact of hypoglycemia unawareness on cognitive dysfunction, Gold et al. (1995) assessed two groups of type 1 diabetic patients (those with normal awareness of hypoglycemia and those without) on a battery of cognitive tests during different conditions of glycemic control. This control was achieved by the use of a glucose clamp. They reported a significant effect of hypoglycemia on cognitive functioning, and a trend for an overall effect of glycemic awareness on a test of Rapid Visual Information Processing (RVIP), across glycemic control conditions. Specifically, in the hypoglycemic condition, the patients who exhibited impaired awareness made more "misses" on the RVIP. Additionally, this group continued to show impaired cognitive functioning on both the Trail Making Test Part B and the RVIP upon recovery of normalized blood glucose levels, suggesting a more lasting effect of hypoglycemia in patients with impaired awareness.

The prevalence of cognitive dysfunction in patients with impaired awareness may also vary with the type of diabetes treatment. For example, Maran et al. (1995) reported that severe hypoglycemia with cognitive dysfunction is three times more common in intensively- rather than conventionally-treated type 1 diabetes. These researches utilized a four choice reaction time measure during euglycemic and hypoglycemic clamping, and reported that deterioration in reaction times occurred at higher glucose levels than did subjective awareness only in intensively-treated patients. Thus, there may be an increased risk of severe hypoglycemia without warning in these intensively-treated patients. Importantly, Fanelli et al. (1997) reported that hypoglycemic unawareness can be reversed by intensive therapy that emphasizes preventing hypoglycemia, suggesting that this regimen has a possible role in the treatment of diabetes-related cognitive dysfunction.

Furthermore, the type of insulin itself may impact the degree of hypoglycemic awareness in some diabetic patients. A reduction in hypoglycemic warning symptoms upon transfer from animal to human insulin formulations has been reported in a subset of diabetic patients (Hepburn et al., 1989; Teuscher & Berger, 1987). In addition, a greater number of sympathoadrenergic symptoms and noradrenaline responses have been reported with porcine insulin in comparison to human insulin in healthy subjects (Heine et al., 1989). These effects could be due to differences in the physicochemical properties of human and animal insulin, as porcine insulin is more lipophilic than human insulin and may thus have greater blood/brain barrier penetration (Heine et al., 1989). Although not all studies have reported such differences (MacLeod et al., 1996; Ferrer et al., 1992), insulin formulation may constitute an important moderating variable for hypoglycemic unawareness, and may warrant consideration in studies of diabetes-related cognitive dysfunction.

Type of Treatment

As noted above, it has been reported that severe hypoglycemia with cognitive dysfunction is three times more likely to occur in intensively- rather than conventionally-treated type 1 diabetic patients (Maran et al., 1995). In an effort to elucidate the relationship between type of treatment and cognitive dysfunction, Reichard et al. (1991) randomized patients to either intensive or regular treatment for a period of three years. They reported that although the number of hypoglycemic events and adrenergic symptoms changed from baseline, no differences were apparent between the two groups on several measures of neuropsychological functioning over time; there were no signs of deteriorating cognitive function in patients with serious hypoglycemic episodes. Additionally, no relationship was found between neuropsychological impairment and intensity of treatment or the number of hypoglycemic episodes in the Diabetes Control and Complications Trial (DCCT Research Group, 1996). The above studies suggest an equivocal role for type of treatment in the development of diabetes-related cognitive dysfunction.

However, intensive insulin treatment is associated with an increased frequency of hypoglycemic coma (Kramer et al., 1998), and it is possible that there may be residual cognitive deficits following diabetic coma. In an effort to determine this possibility, Kramer et al. (1998) investigated cognitive function and electrophysiological indexes in patients with or without a history of coma and normal control subjects. They reported that despite differences in P300 latencies between patients who had experienced a diabetic coma and healthy control subjects (which correlated with duration of illness), no relationship was seen between electrophysiological measures and the presence of hypoglycemic coma. Additionally, MMSE and Trail Making test scores did not differ between diabetic patients with a history of coma and control subjects. Furthermore, previous episodes of hypoglycemic coma were not associated with any permanent impairment of cognitive function (when comparing subjects with or without a history of coma). As in prior studies, cognitive functioning was impaired only in relation to duration of illness. These studies suggest that type of treatment in itself, or history of diabetic coma, may not be very critical in the genesis or maintenance of cognitive dysfunction in type 1 diabetes.

Polyneuropathy

There has been some suggestion that the psychomotor slowing seen in prior neuropsychological investigations of diabetic patients may be more attributable to polyneuropathy than true central dysfunction, as many of the tests that discriminated diabetic from control patients had a motor component. Ryan et al. (1992) reported that the presence of distal symmetric polyneuropathy was strongly associated with psychomotor slowing, and that glycated hemoglobin was relatively less associated with psychomotor slowing and spatial processing. In a later study, Ryan et al. (1993) reported that the best biomedical predictor of cognitive performance in a group of diabetic subjects was a diagnosis of polyneuropathy. Although these researchers failed to find an effect for recurrent hypoglycemia, they did report an interaction between episodes of hypoglycemia and the presence of neuropathy, suggesting that recurrent hypoglycemia may interact with neuropathy to exaggerate the extent of neuropsychological dysfunction seen in diabetic patients.

However, other studies have failed to find such a relationship. In a group of relatively younger patients (aged less than 55) with type 2 diabetes, Dey et al. (1997) reported that although more patients had impaired performance on Neurobehavioral Cognitive Status Examination measures of attention, repetition, and memory than demographically-matched, normal control subjects, the presence of distal polyneuropathy did not correlate with performance on these measures.

Presence of Lacunae

It is widely accepted that diabetes can interfere with cognitive functioning indirectly through relatively large cerebrovascular events such as frank infarcts. However, the relationship between smaller asymptomatic cerebral infarcts (lacunae) and cognitive function in diabetes is largely unknown. In an effort to elucidate this relationship, Fushimi (1996) reported that among type 2 diabetic patients, 42% showed evidence of infarcts or lacunae on MRI. The incidence of lacunae was significantly higher in older patients but was not related to other risk factors for atherosclerosis. Importantly, the presence of lacunae was correlated with age, intellectual ability, and spatial cognitive ability (cube drawing). However, a significant correlation between cube drawing impairment and lacunae was also seen in the non-diabetic patient group, suggesting that the presence of lacunae may be an important but nonspecific variable in diabetes-related cognitive impairment.

Blood Pressure

In a prospective study of 187 type 2 diabetic patients and 1624 healthy control subjects followed for 28–30 years (Framingham study), Elias et al. (1997) revealed that the presence and duration of type 2 diabetes and blood pressure interacted in such a way as to result in decreased performance on measures of visual memory and composite neuropsychological functioning (composed of eight measures of learning, memory, visual organization, verbal fluency, concept formation, and abstract reasoning). Additionally, the duration of type 2 diabetes was associated with poorer performance on measures of verbal memory and concept formation. Finally, insulin-treated patients with type 2 diabetes were reported to be at higher risk for poor neuropsychological test performance than those controlled with diet or oral agents.

Depression

The presence of depression is known to be associated with increased cognitive complaints, and can adversely affect objective cognitive function in a variety of patients, especially on measures of psychomotor speed and complex attention. Not surprisingly, in patients with type 2 diabetes, a trend has also been noted for increased self-reported levels of depression and memory problems (Tun et al., 1987). Additionally, heightened depression has been associated with various indicators of neuropathy, and with significant reductions in self-regulated control of glucose. Depression therefore should be considered an important variable in the assessment of diabetes-related cognitive dysfunction. Unfortunately, there have been very few published studies investigating the role of depression in the development and maintenance of cognitive impairment in diabetes.

In one such population-based study of 80 diabetic and 81 non-diabetic Native Americans, Lowe et al. (1994) reported that type 2 diabetes was associated with impairment on a measure of verbal fluency. However, they reported that the difference between the two groups on this measure could be accounted for by differences in depression, hypertension, and alcohol use. Other studies have investigated the relationship between depression and other symptoms of diabetes. For example, Geringer et al. (1988) failed to find any significant linear or quadratic relationship between peripheral neuropathy and self-reported depression scores (Zung Self-Rating Depression Scale) in diabetic women. However, they did report a significant relationship between depression and objective measurements of peripheral neuropathy in women with scores over 50, suggesting that moderate depression is more likely to be seen in patients who have peripheral neuropathy. Additionally, Lustman et al. (1988) reported that self-reported depression (Beck Depression Inventory) was moderately correlated with numerous diabetes symptoms, and had a significant effect on the reporting of both hyperglycemia and hypoglycemic symptoms, as well as nonspecific symptoms of poor metabolic control. It is possible that many of the reported symptoms often attributed to poor diabetic control (e.g., impaired short-term memory and reduced psychomotor speed) are more closely related to depression than metabolic control. Thus, diabetic symptoms may be unreliable indicators of poor metabolic control in depressed patients.

Ethnicity

In a comparison of the clinical features and vascular complications of diabetes between 456 Caucasians and 451 Asians, Samanta et al. (1991) reported that Asians were less likely to have peripheral vascular disease (3.7% vs. 9.3%) and retinopathy (11.6% vs. 32.3%) than Caucasians, but were more likely to have renal disease (22.3% vs. 12.6%). These differences remained after adjustments for age, sex, duration of diabetes, age at onset, hypertension, smoking, treatment with insulin, body mass index, or physical activity levels. As cognitive complaints are often associated with the presence of retinopathy and nephropathy, the incidence of cognitive dysfunction may also vary significantly among certain ethnic subgroups that differ in the prevalence of diabetes-related complications. Additional studies examining the prevalence of diabetes-related cognitive dysfunction in various ethnic groups are necessary to assess the impact of race and ethnicity on this disorder.

STRATEGIES IN THE MEASUREMENT AND ANALYSIS OF NEUROPSYCHOLOGICAL FUNCTIONING

Upon successful quantification and experimental control of the various modifying variables and risk factors listed above, the next step to help ensure successful completion of a trial designed to assess diabetes-related cognitive dysfunction is to utilize the appropriate neuropsychological instruments that are sensitive to treatment effects. There are numerous individual neuropsychological tests that have been shown to be sensitive in distinguishing diabetic from non-diabetic patients, as well as in detecting cognitive changes associated with treatment. However, given the multitude of assessment possibilities proposed in the literature, it is difficult to select the exact neuropsychological measure or measures that will accomplish the specified goal of the study. Some clinicians and researchers have promoted the use of a fixed battery approach like the Luria Nebraska (Golden et al., 1980) or the Halstead-Reitan (Reitan and Wolfson, 1985), which provide comprehensive coverage of multiple neuropsychological domains. However, these batteries are very lengthy to administer and have not yielded convincing results in the diabetes literature. Conversely, a single test approach may not adequately probe the discrete cognitive dysfunction seen in this patient group. One difficulty with past research that has highlighted the significance of an exclusive cognitive deficit (e.g., involving memory) in various patient populations is that the design only allowed for one cognitive domain to be measured. Put in other words, the probability of finding memory deficits in a given patient significantly increases when only tests of memory are given. Although this single domain approach certainly saves time, these studies cannot accurately assess the degree of memory dysfunction in relation to other areas of cognition dysfunction and cognitive sparing. Thus, there is a tradeoff between time spent on each assessment procedure and the amount of information needed to make correct and valid generalizations regarding treatment effects. Given this tradeoff, a comprehensive battery of cognitive tests designed to assess several selective neuropsychological functions might prove optimal in identifying and tracking cognitive dysfunction in this patient population.

To aid in this approach, the use of composite neuropsychological summary scales constructed to encompass various neuropsychological domains of functioning (e.g., frontal attention, motor attention, and verbal and spatial memory) is recommended. The composition of summary scales should reflect both current neuropsychological research and theory on diabetes. Additionally, scale construction should attempt to reflect the known neuroanatomical literature regarding the functional geography of the brain. For example, spatial memory measures should be employed that are known to be sensitive to right hemisphere lesions. In this way, the cognitive deficits associated with diabetes could be lateralized or localized in a manner that will better help researchers and clinicians understand the pathophysiology underlying this disorder.

The use of such summary scales also helps to control for the large Type I error inherent in collecting multiple dependent measures, as seen with various neuropsychological procedures. In fact, some individual memory tests may have as many as 25 different dependent variables providing a separate metric for each learning trial (e.g., an overall learning curve, percent retention, signal detection variables, and scores for each condition such as short and long delays, cued recall, and free recall).

Although every neuropsychological test obviously taps multiple cognitive domains (e.g., all tests measure attention to some degree) it is possible to characterize most neuropsychological tests into one or two discrete categories that reflect a singular primary cognitive construct such as verbal memory or visual organization. Outlined below are some examples of various neuropsychological summary scales that were designed for a diabetes study, and the constituent individual neuropsychological tests (with salient metrics) utilized in their construction. For more information on these and other specific neuropsychological tests, their psychometric proprieties, and their relation to functional neuroanatomy, please refer to Lezak (1995).

1. *Attention Scale:* This scale includes the number of correct responses from the Reaction Time, Vigilance, and Distraction Portions of the computerized Continuous Performance Test (CPT) from Gordon Diagnostic Systems (Gordon, 1986). The first test (Reaction time) measures the subject's ability to respond to a number when flashed on the screen. The Vigilance portion requires more complex attentional skills, in which the subject must respond to a number that is followed by another number. The Distraction condition utilizes the same strategy as the Vigilance condition, but distractor numbers are added in other screen columns. The total time to complete Trail Making Test Part A (Army Individual Test Battery, 1944), a measure of simple attention and motor speed, can also be utilized in this summary scale.

2. *Executive Functioning Scale:* This scale includes the number of correct categories achieved on the Wisconsin Card Sort (WCST; Heaton, 1981). With this measure of frontal lobe functioning, patients must match cards on one of three possible conceptual categories and be able to switch cognitive sets throughout the test. The number of words generated on the Controlled Oral Word Association (COWA) test (Benton and Hamsher, 1978), a test of phonemic verbal fluency as well as animal naming (semantic fluency), both of which are thought to be sensitive to frontal lobe lesions, is also included. The total time spent completing the Trail Making Test Part B (Army Individual Test Battery, 1944), which measures a subject's ability to shift cognitive sets between letters and numbers, can be used, as well as the number of correctly identified colors on the interference portion of the Stroop Color-Word Test (Golden, 1978).

3. *Verbal Memory Scale:* This scale was constructed with the following neuropsychological scores: total scores on the Semantic Prose portions of the Wechsler Memory Scale Revised (WMS-R, Wechsler, 1987) subtests for both immediate and 30-minute delayed recall conditions, the total number of items recalled on the fifth trial, the total after all five trial presentations, and the number of items recalled on the 20-minute delayed recognition portion of the California Verbal Learning Test (CVLT; DeLis,

1987). Finally, the number of correctly identified words on the Low-Imagery Word Recognition Memory Test, in which subjects must identify 20 previously viewed low-imagery words from a group of 40 abstract words in both an immediate and delayed condition (30 minutes later), was also included.

4. ***Spatial Memory Scale:*** This scale was developed using the following measures: total score on the Visual Design portion of the WMS-R subtests for both immediate and 30-minute delayed recall conditions, and the number of correctly identified faces on the Facial Memory Recognition Memory Test in both immediate and delayed conditions. In this test, the subject must correctly identify a group of 20 faces (taken from a yearbook) from a group of 40 faces.

In addition to the above neuropsychological scales reflecting specific cognitive domains, it is possible to construct more global scales based on cerebral lateralization. For example, a scale reflecting ***Right Hemisphere*** functioning can be constructed that consists of all of the items on the Spatial Memory Scale; the score on the Block Design subtest of the Wechsler Adult Intelligence Scale-Revised version (WAIS-R); the number correct on the Benton Line Orientation Scale (Benton, Hamsher, Varney and Spreen, 1983), in which subjects must match lines of similar orientation and position to a model; and the scores on the Drawing to Command and Copy subtests (Saykin et al., 1995), in which subjects must copy or draw geometric figures.

Similarly, the ***Left Hemisphere Scale*** can be constructed utilizing all measures from the Verbal Memory scales, as well as measures of both receptive and expressive language. These include the total naming score on the Boston Naming Test (Kaplan et al., 1978) and the number of correctly answered questions on the Comprehension of Complex Ideational Material Test, in which subjects are read short paragraphs and must answer "yes" or "no" to statements concerning these paragraphs. These measures are subtests of the Boston Diagnostic Aphasia Exam (Goodglass and Kaplan, 1983). The number correct on the Modified Token Test (Benton and Hamsher, 1978), in which subjects must manipulate different colored chips according to simple and complex oral commands (Goodglass and Kaplan, 1983), can also be used. Finally, this scale can also include the number of correctly repeated sentences on the Benton Repetition Test (Benton and Hamsher, 1978). The two latter measures are part of the Multilingual Aphasia Battery.

Neuropsychological summary scales must be constructed by first converting all raw individual scores to a common metric. This can be accomplished by using age-appropriate normative means and standard deviations from normal healthy control subjects that are already published or attained during the actual investigation. Calculating Z scores based on these norms allows for easy compilation across tests by providing a common and normalized metric. This technique also allows for the use of regression-based corrections for gender, age, and premorbid intellectual functioning (Saykin et al. 1995), all of which are important in neuropsychological research. The use of tests with comparable psychometric properties is important in establishing a differential deficit in schizophrenia and is necessary when attempting to support a selective area of impairment (Chapman and Chapman, 1989). Z scores within each neuropsychological summary scale can then be averaged to achieve a single Z score reflecting the average level of performance on a given summary scale (i.e., Spatial Memory), and can even be weighted differently based on *a priori* hypotheses. For more detail on the actual construction of various composite summary scales, refer to

Riordan et al. (1999) or Saykin et al. (1995). Utilizing summary scales allows for ease of comparison across cognitive domains or in making laterality comparisons. It also allows for the easy comparison of cognitive domains across time and treatment conditions. Changes in Z scores of at least one standard deviation can serve as an adequate threshold for assessing clinically meaningful diversity over time that may be due to treatment. Additionally, normative composite test measures may serve as surrogate markers for true biologic endpoints.

To function as a surrogate marker, cognitive variables must have sound biological, epidemiological, and statistical bases (Donald and Weihrauch, 1998). Establishing the validity of the cognitive marker also requires a known relationship between surrogate and clinical endpoints. Additionally, these markers should be fairly convenient (i.e., easily obtainable) and the anticipated clinical benefit should be deducible from changes in the surrogate marker. Some examples of accepted and validated surrogate endpoints include blood pressure for stroke, cholesterol for cardiac survival, and HbA_{1c} for reduction of microvascular complications. Composite cognitive variables such as those presented above appear to meet the criteria for valid surrogate makers, and may eventually serve as surrogates for various biological indicators of hypoglycemic response in clinical trials of experimentally-controlled glycemia and in controlled trial settings.

TREATMENT STRATEGIES

Patients with chronic illnesses often report that their most bothersome symptom is cognitive in nature, despite the apparent severity of their physical difficulties. Cognitive clarity is considered to be an extremely important issue in quality of life for almost all chronic patient groups, which underscores the importance of addressing cognitive concerns in many patient populations. It is therefore surprising that more studies have not included objective cognitive measures when assessing treatment effects in diabetes.

One randomized, double-blind study that assessed the role of subjective cognitive dysfunction in type 2 diabetes was conducted by Testa and Simonson (1998), who reported significant quality of life treatment differences, including general perceived health and cognitive functioning, between patients undergoing active therapy with glipizide extended release tablets (Glucotrol XL®) and those receiving placebo. Specifically, subscales reflecting sleep and depression (both of which relate to cognitive functioning) were the most affected by treatment. They concluded that subjective cognitive dysfunction was apparent in these diabetic patients, and that this subjective cognitive dysfunction responded positively to short-term antidiabetic treatment.

In a similar trial of glycemic control conducted in older patients with type 2 diabetes, Gradman et al. (1993) reported that improved glycemic control resulted in improvements in objective learning and memory with glipizide treatment. Specifically, this improvement was apparent in the encoding of verbal material. No changes were seen in measures of attention and complex perceptual-motor function, and as expected, simple perceptual-motor functioning did not show any improvement with treatment. Another study of elderly type 2 diabetic patients (Naor et al., 1997) reported that psychomotor speed and concentration improved after inpatient treatment for metabolic control. This improvement was maintained and actually enhanced 6 weeks after discharge from the treatment program.

This study suggests that cognitive deficits in elderly type 2 diabetic patients can be reduced despite the lack of benefits on other dependent measures. Results from these few studies indicate that both subjective and various aspects of objective cognitive functioning can improve with improved glycemic control, and that these improvements may outlast the experimental treatment.

CONCLUSIONS

A large and growing body of evidence supports the assumption that central nervous system dysfunction exists in patients with diabetes, and is often expressed as mild cognitive impairment. However, not all studies have confirmed this assumption. For example, in a review of 19 published, controlled studies on type 2 diabetes and cognitive dysfunction, Strachan (1997) found that only 13 studies reported that diabetic patients performed more poorly than control subjects on at least one aspect of cognitive function. The remaining six studies showed no differences. It is important to note that none of these six studies had adequate statistical power to detect between-group differences for a medium effect size of 0.5 standard deviations. This underpowering of studies results from the small effect sizes anticipated in this disorder (i.e., the level of cognitive impairment is usually mild).

Nonetheless, the overwhelming majority of studies suggest that the CNS manifestations of diabetes are expressed in measures of higher cognitive abilities, rather than simple motor function. This suggests that the differences seen between diabetic patients and control groups on neuropsychological measures cannot be explained by the presence of peripheral neuropathy alone. Furthermore, cognitive abnormalities are more likely to be expressed during the performance of complex neuropsychological measures, rather than simple ones. For example, cognitive deficits are more likely to be seen on complex measures of attention that involve vigilance, working memory, and psychomotor speed, rather than on measures of simple reaction time. The notion that more challenging tasks are necessary to allow observation of these deficits is consistent with a prior cerebral blood flow (CBF) study by Dandona et al. (1978), who challenged diabetic patients and control subjects with inhalation of 5% CO_2. Under this condition, 86% of control subjects exhibited increased CBF in comparison to only 39% of diabetic patients. In other words, when the metabolic demand of the brain was increased, the diabetic patients did not respond with a normal increase in CBF. Mechanisms that account for this observation likely impact neuropsychological assessment procedures. This understanding may help to explain why diabetic patients seem to have relatively intact performance on simple motor and attentional tasks, but are impaired in more demanding measures of memory and executive functioning.

Additionally, two separate but possibly related patterns of test performance have consistently emerged from the above reviewed literature on cognitive dysfunction in diabetes. These patterns of cognitive dysfunction suggest that while diabetic patients appear to perform worse than normal control subjects on many cognitive measures, they appear to have a selective deficit in measures of visual spatial and executive functioning. This suggests that central manifestations of diabetes may be more prominent in the right hemisphere and frontal-subcortical system. It is important to note that the selective deficit in visual measures could not be accounted for by retinopathy in these patients. The reasons for lateralized and localized effects on the brain in diabetes are presently unknown. Regions involved in frontal-subcortical circuitry possibly may be more prone to damage caused by hypoglycemia, in much the same way that these structures are more susceptible to the adverse effects of hypoxia or carbon monoxide exposure. The preponderance of right hemisphere deficits is more difficult to explain, but may partially be due to the relatively disproportionate involvement of the right hemisphere in attentional function.

The relationship between diabetes and cognitive dysfunction is mediated by numerous biological/psychosocial variables and various risk factors. The most important variables associated with the presence of cognitive dysfunction in diabetes appear to be duration of illness, presence of severe hypoglycemic episodes, and presence of neuropathy. However, it is also important to note that the interaction of these moderating variables may actually be more important in the presentation of cognitive dysfunction in diabetes than the effect of any one variable alone. For example, although no direct relationship between type of treatment and cognitive dysfunction has been consistently reported, the interaction between type of treatment and hypoglycemic unawareness has been shown to adversely affect cognitive functioning. Additionally, there may be additive effects when two variables known to adversely impact cognitive function are present and interact. For example, it is possible that recurrent hypoglycemia may interact with neuropathy to exaggerate the extent of neuropsychological dysfunction seen in patients with type 1 diabetes.

Unfortunately, comprehensive and careful examination of cognitive dysfunction in diabetes has yet to be conducted in controlled clinical trials. This is disappointing given the prevalence of cognitive dysfunction often seen in this patient population, the importance that patients assign to cognition in their quality of life, and the close relationship between neuropsychological and various biological makers of this disease. Sensitive composite measures of cognitive functioning may possibly serve as a surrogate maker for more substantial, long-term clinical benefits. Such measures could help to enhance the estimated benefit-to-risk relationship of therapies aimed at other diabetic outcomes. Conceivably, better characterization of diabetes-induced CNS disease and the validation of surrogate endpoints could enable the pursuit of CNS therapeutic indications. The best chance of finding such a measure is in including valid and reliable composite neuropsychological summary scales in large interventional or observational trials. Finally, this review suggests not only the utility of cognitive markers in the assessment of treatment response to antidiabetic agents, but points to a role for therapeutic agents in the amelioration of cognitive decline seen in patients with type 1 and type 2 diabetes.

References

Army Individual Test Battery. *Manual of Directions and Scoring.* Washington, D.C., War Dept. Adjutant General's Office, 1944.

Benton A, Hamsher K, Varney N, Spreen O. *Contributions to Neuropsychological Assessment.* New York: Oxford University Press, 1983.

Benton A, Hamsher K. *Multilingual Aphasia Examination.* Iowa City: University of Iowa Press, 1978.

Chapman L, Chapman J. Strategies for resolving the heterogeneity of schizophrenics and their relatives using cognitive measures. *J Abnorm Psychol* 1989, **98**(4): 357–366.

Cox DJ, Gonder-Frederick LA, Schroeder DB, Cryer PE, Clarke WL. Disruptive effects of acute hypoglycemia on speed of cognitive and motor performance. *Diabetes Care* 1993; **16**(10): 1391–1393.

Croxson SC, Jagger C. Diabetes and cognitive impairment: a community-based study of elderly subjects. *Age Ageing* 1995; **24**(5): 421–424.

Dandona P, James I, Newbury P, Woollard MC, Beckett AG. Cerebral blood flow in diabetes mellitus: evidence for cerebrovascular reactivity. *BMJ* 1978; **2**: 325–326.

DCCT Research Group. Effects of intensive diabetes therapy on neuropsychological function in adults in the Diabetes Control and Complications Trial. *Ann Intern Med* 1996; **124**(4): 379–388.

DeLis D, Kramer J, Kaplan E. *California Verbal Learning Test: Research edition.* San Antonio: Psychological Corporation, 1987.

Dey J, Misra A, Desai NG, Mahapatra AK, Padma MV. Cognitive function in younger type II diabetes. *Diabetes Care* 1997; **20**(1): 32–35.

Donald P, Weihrauch R. Surrogate endpoints: their utility for evaluating therapeutic effect in clinical trials. *App Clin Trials* 1998; **7**(10): 46–56.

Draelos MT, Jacobson AM, Weinger K, Widom B, Ryan CM, Finkelstein DM, Simonson DC. (1995). Cognitive function in patients with insulin-dependant diabetes mellitus during hyperglycemia and hypoglycemia. *Am J Med* 1995; **98**(2): 135–144.

Elias PK, Elias MF, D'Agostino RB, Cupples LA, Wilson PW, Silbershatz H, Wolf PA. NIDDM and blood pressure as risk factors for poor cognitive performance. The Framingham Study. *Diabetes Care* 1997; **20**(9): 1388–1395.

Fanelli C, Pampanelli S, Lalli C, Del Sindaco P, Ciofetta M, Lepore M, Porcellati F, Bottini P, Di Vincenzo A, Brunetti P, et al. Long-term intensive therapy of IDDM patients with clinically overt autonomic neuropathy: effects of hypoglycemia awareness and counterregulation. *Diabetes* 1997; **46**(7): 1172–1181.

Ferrer JP, Esmatjes E, Gonzalez-Clemente JM, Goday A, Conget I, Jiminez W, Gomis R, Rivera F, Vilardell E. Symptomatic and hormonal hypoglycaemic responses to human and porcine insulin in patients with type 1 diabetes mellitus. *Diabet Med* 1992; **9**(6): 522–527.

Fushimi H, Inoue T, Yamada Y, Udaka F, Kameyama M. Asymptomatic cerebral small infarcts (lacunae), their risk factors and intellectual disturbances. *Diabetes* 1996; **45**(Suppl 3): S98–100.

Geringer ES, Perlmuter LC, Stern TA, Nathan DM. Depression and diabetic neuropathy: a complex relationship. *J Geriatr Psychiatry Neurol* 1988, **1**(1): 11–15.

Gold AE, MacLeod KM, Deary IJ, Frier BM. Hypoglycemia-induced cognitive dysfunction in diabetes mellitus: effect of hypoglycemia unawareness. *Physiol Behav* 1995; **58**(3): 501–511.

Golden C. *Stroop Color and Word Test.* Chicago: Stoelting Co, 1978.

Golden C, Hammeke T, Purisch A. *Luria Nebraska Neuropsychology Battery (manual).* Los Angeles: Western Psychological Services, 1980.

Goodglass H, Kaplan E. *The Assessment of Aphasia and Related Disorders: Second Edition.* Philadelphia: Lea and Febiger, 1983.

Gordon M. *The Gordon Diagnostic System.* Dewitt, NY: Gordon Systems Inc., 1986.

Gradman TJ, Laws A, Thompson LW, Reaven GM. Verbal learning and/or memory improves with glycemic control in older subjects with non-insulin-dependant diabetes mellitus. *J Am Geriatr Soc* 1993; **41**(12): 305–312.

Haeton R. *The Wisconsin Card Sorting Test.* New York: Psychological Assessment Resources, 1981.

Heine RJ, van der Heyden EA, van der Veen EA. Responses to human and porcine insulin in healthy subjects. *Lancet* 1989; **2**(8669): 946–949.

Hepburn DA, Eadington DW, Patrick AW, Colledge NR, Frier BM. Symptomatic awareness of hypoglycemia: does it change on transfer from animal to human insulin? *Diabet Med* 1989; **6**(7): 586–590.

Hershey T, Craft S, Bhargava N, White NH. Memory and insulin dependant diabetes mellitus (IDDM): effects of childhood onset and severe hypoglycemia. *J Int Neuropsychol Soc* 1997; **3**(6): 509–520.

Hoffman RG, Speelman DJ, Hinnen DA, Conley KL, Guthrie RA, Knapp RK. Changes in cortical functioning with acute hypoglycemia and hyperglycemia in type I diabetes. *Diabetes Care* 1989; **12**(3): 193–197.

Kaplan E, Goodglass H, Weintraub S. *The Boston Naming Test.* Philadelphia: Lea and Febiger, 1978.

Kramer L, Fasching P, Madl C, Schneider B, Damjancic P, Waldhausl W, Irsigler K, Grimm G. Previous episodes of hypoglycemic coma are not associated with permanent cognitive brain dysfunction in IDDM patients on intensive insulin treatment. *Diabetes* 1998, **47**(12): 1909–1914.

L'Hommedieu A, Podraza AM. A bibliography of the neurobehavioral aspects of diabetes mellitus. *Exp Aging Res* 1989; **15**(3-4): 203–205.

Langan SJ, Deary IJ, Hepburn DA, Frier BM. Cumulative cognitive impairment following recurrent severe hypoglycaemia in adult patients with insulin-treated diabetes mellitus. *Diabetologia* 1991; **34**(5): 337–344.

Lezak, M. *Neuropsychological Assessment: Third Edition.* New York: Oxford University Press, 1995.

Lincoln NB, Faleiro RM, Kelly C, Kirk BA, Jeffcoate WJ. Effect of long-term glycemic control on cognitive function. *Diabetes Care* 1996; **19**(6): 656–658.

Lowe LP, Tranel D, Wallace RB, Welty TK. Type II diabetes and cognitive function. A population-based study of Native Americans. *Diabetes Care* 1994; **17**(8): 891–898.

Lustman PJ, Clouse RE, Carney RM. Depression and the reporting of diabetes symptoms. *Int J Psychiatry Med* 1988; **18**(4): 295–303.

MacLeod KM, Gold AE, Frier BM. A comparative study of responses to acute hypoglycaemia induced by human and porcine insulins in patients with type 1 diabetes. *Diabet Med* 1996; **13**(4): 346–357.

Maran A., Lomas J, Macdonald IA, Amiel SA. Lack of preservation of higher brain function during hypoglycaemia in patients with intensively-treated IDDM. *Diabetologia* 1995; **38**(12): 1412–1418.

Messier C, Gagnon M. Glucose regulation and cognitive functions: relation to Alzheimer's disease and diabetes. *Behav Brain Res* 1996; **75**(1-2): 1–11.

Mooradian AD. Pathophysiology of central nervous system complications in diabetes mellitus. *Clin Neurosci* 1997; **4**(6): 322–326.

Naor M, Steingruber HJ, Westhoff K, Schottenfeld-Naor Y, Gries AF. Cognitive function in elderly non-insulin-dependent diabetic patients before and after inpatient treatment for metabolic control. *J Diabetes Complications* 1997; **11**(1): 40–46.

Ott A, Stolk RP, Hofman A, van Harskamp F, Grobbee DE, Breteler MM. Association of diabetes mellitus and dementia: the Rotterdam Study. *Diabetologia* 1996, **39**(11): 1392–1397.

Prescott JH, Richardson JT, Gillespie CR. Cognitive function in diabetes mellitus: the effects of duration of illness and glycaemic control. *Br J Clin Psychol* 1990; **29**(Pt 2): 167–175.

Reichard P, Berglund A, Britz A, Levander S, Rosenqvist U. Hypoglycemic episodes during intensified insulin treatment: increased frequency but no effect on cognitive function. *J Intern Med* 1991; **229**(1): 9–16.

Reitan R, Wolfson D. *The Halstead-Reitan Neuropsychological Test Battery: Theory and Clinical Interpretation.* Tucson, AZ: Neuropsychology Press, 1985.

Riordan H, Flashman L, Saykin A, Frutiger S, Carroll K, Huey L. Neuropsychological correlates of methylphenidate treatment in adult ADHD with and without depression. *Arch Clin Neuropsych* 1999; **14**(2): 217–233.

Ryan CM. Neurobehavioral complications of type I diabetes. Examination of possible risk factors. *Diabetes Care* 1988; **11**(1): 86–93.

Ryan CM, Williams TM, Finegold DN, Orchard TJ. Cognitive dysfunction in adults with type 1 (insulin-dependant) diabetes mellitus of long duration: effects of recurrent hypoglycaemia and other chronic complications. *Diabetologia* 1993; **36**(4): 329–334.

Ryan CM, Williams TM, Orchard TJ, Finegold DN. Psychomotor slowing is associated with distal symmetrical polyneuropathy in adults with diabetes mellitus. *Diabetes* 1992; **41**(1): 107–113.

Samanta A, Burden AC, Jagger C. A comparison of the clinical features and vascular complications of diabetes between migrant Asians and Caucasians in Leicester, U.K. *Diabetes Res Clin Pract* 1991; **14**(3): 205–213.

Saykin A, Gur RC, Gur RE, Shtasel D, Flannery K, Mozley L, Robinson L, Malamut B, Watson BJ, Mozely D. Normative neuropsychological test performance: effects of age, education, gender, ethnicity. *Applied Neuropsychology* 1995; **2**: 79–88.

Strachan MW, Deary IJ, Ewing FM, Frier BM. Is type II diabetes associated with an increased risk of cognitive dysfunction? A critical review of published studies. *Diabetes Care* 1997; **20**(3): 438–445.

Testa MA, Simonson DC. Health economic benefits and quality of life during improved glycemic control in patients with type 2 diabetes mellitus: a randomized, controlled, double-blind trial. *JAMA* 1998; **280**(17): 1490–1496.

Teuscher A, Berger WG. Hypoglycaemia unawareness in diabetics transferred from beef/porcine insulin to human insulin. *Lancet* 1987; **2**(8555): 382–385.

Tun PA, Perlmuter LC, Russo P, Nathan DM. Memory self-assessment and performance in aged diabetics and non-diabetics. *Exp Aging Res* 1987; **13**(3): 151–157.

Wechsler D. *Wecshler Memory Scale Revised Manual.* San Antonio, TX: The Psychological Corporation, 1987.

Wredling R, Levander S, Adamson U, Lins PE. Permanent neuropsychological impairment after recurrent episodes of severe hypoglycaemia in man. *Diabetologia* 1990; **33**(3): 152–157.

Ziegler D, Langen KJ, Herzog H, Kuwert T, Muhlen H, Feinendegen LE, Gries FA. Cerebral glucose metabolism in type 1 diabetic patients. *Diabet Med* 1994; **11**(2): 205–209.

12

SPECIAL METHODOLOGICAL CONSIDERATIONS

There are some special methodological considerations in the development of antidiabetic therapies which warrant further discussion. Specifically, two types of study designs, in addition to those required for regulatory approval, may contribute to the optimization of a therapeutic development plan. In this chapter, the use of early exploratory studies to optimize dosing and reduce development time, as well as the growing role of pharmacoeconomic studies in clinical drug development, will be discussed.

THE ROLE OF THE BRIDGING STUDY IN DRUG DEVELOPMENT

The timely completion of a drug development program is dependent upon the selection of an appropriate dose range for clinical evaluation. A standard approach for first-in-human (Phase I) studies is to select a dose range based on animal toxicity findings, and to assess the safety and tolerability of this range in samples of healthy subjects. Based on the results in healthy subjects, doses are then revised for later efficacy studies in the patient population. The use of healthy populations, rather than patients, in these initial studies has several advantages, including both convenience and safety (Weissman, 1981). However, extensive evidence has indicated that the safety and tolerability of numerous compounds differ substantially between patients and healthy subjects. Thus, dose-finding studies in a healthy population may be poorly predictive of the optimal dose range for efficacy trials in patients.

Significant differences in tolerance between healthy and patient populations have previously been observed with compounds for the treatment of Alzheimer's disease, schizophrenia, anxiety, and depression (reviewed in Cutler et al., 1998; Murphy et al., 1998; Sramek et al., 1997; Cutler et al., 1996; Cutler et al., 1994). These differences are not entirely surprising, as these drug classes are designed to affect underlying factors (e.g., neurotransmitters, receptors, etc.) that are altered in the disease state. Antidiabetic compounds, which target abnormalities in metabolic function, are also likely to affect patients and healthy subjects differently. For example, the occurrence of hypoglycemia, the most commonly reported adverse event with antidiabetic drugs, is likely to emerge at different doses in subjects with normal insulin activity than in diabetic patients with a relative insulin deficiency. In addition, the pharmacokinetic properties of a compound may be affected by factors associated with diabetes, such as delayed gastric emptying due to autonomic neuropathy, or renal insufficiency due to nephropathy.

For compounds that exert maximal efficacy at the high end of the tolerability spectrum, the failure to determine an optimal range prior to large-scale efficacy trials can result in ambiguous data if the selected doses are too low, or excessive toxicity if the doses are too high (Figure 12.1). Many antidiabetic therapies have demonstrated significant dose-response effects for efficacy or adverse events, including metformin (Garber et al., 1997), acarbose (Fischer et al., 1998), miglitol (Scott & Tattersall, 1988), and glimepiride (Goldberg et al., 1996), suggesting that the selection of accurate doses is of particular importance for this therapeutic class.

In order to address differences between patients and healthy subjects that may affect optimal dosing, the bridging study has been developed (Cutler et al., 1996; Cutler and Sramek, 1998, 1995). The bridging study is a late Phase I or early Phase II safety/tolerance study designed to determine the maximum tolerated dose (MTD) of a compound in the target patient population, prior to the initiation of efficacy trials. Dose ranges for Phase II efficacy studies are thus based on results obtained in patients, rather than observations in healthy subjects. The inclusion of a bridging study in a development program can help to avoid the delays and costs associated with adjusting the dose range after efficacy trials have begun (Figure 12.2).

Methodology of the Bridging Study

In a bridging study, consecutive panels of 6–8 patients (4–6 active drug, 2 placebo) receive rising, fixed doses of the investigational compound until a minimum intolerated dose

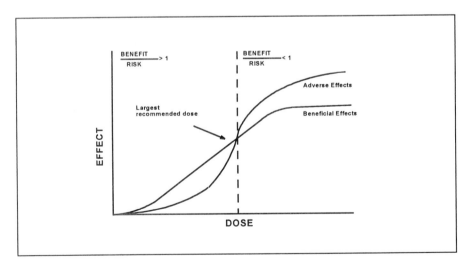

Figure 12.1 - Example of a dose-response curve for adverse and beneficial effects. From Cutler et al., 1998. Copyright John Wiley & Sons Limited. Reproduced with permission.

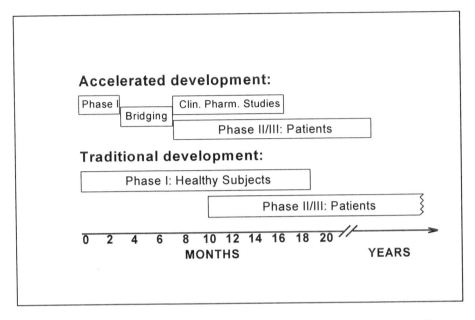

Figure 12.2 - Timelines for accelerated versus traditional therapeutic development. From Cutler et al., 1998. Copyright John Wiley & Sons Limited. Reproduced with permission.

(MID) is reached. The MID is defined as the dose at which 50% of the patients in a panel experience severe or multiple moderate adverse events that are judged to be probably related to the study drug, or one patient experiences a serious adverse event (defined as medically unacceptable) that is judged to be related to the study drug. The dose immediately below the MID is designated the MTD (Cutler et al., 1997). Fixed doses for bridging study panels generally range from 50% below to 50% above the MTD determined in healthy subjects. If the MTD in healthy subjects has not been determined, then the maximum dose for the bridging study is based on the No Toxic Effect Level observed in preclinical studies. In addition to the fixed dose panels, a final panel may be included to assess titration of the investigational compound. In some cases, there may be differences in tolerability between fixed and titrated doses, and titration could redefine the MTD or identify a more optimal dosing regimen (Cutler and Sramek, 1998).

As bridging studies necessarily explore doses at the high end of the tolerability spectrum, these studies are conducted in an inpatient setting with hospital-quality intensive care equipment, under the close supervision of qualified critical care nurses and physicians. In addition, patients are required to be in good physical health (other than the target indication), with no significant concomitant medical disease. Patients are frequently questioned about negative experiences throughout the study, to assure that adverse events do not go unreported.

Bridging studies can enhance the efficiency of the drug development process by ensuring that the relevant dose range is identified as early as possible. By optimizing the design of later efficacy trials, bridging studies can also maximize the potential to identify effective new antidiabetic therapies.

PHARMACOECONOMIC APPROACHES IN DRUG DEVELOPMENT

With the growth of managed care in the U.S., pharmacoeconomic studies are likely to become a more common aspect of drug development. There are several types of pharmacoeconomic studies, which can be distinguished by the factors that are compared to the net cost of the therapy. While a *cost-minimization* analysis compares only the net cost of the therapy with that of alternative therapies, a *cost-effectiveness* analysis evaluates both the clinical consequences (e.g., years of life saved) and net costs of alternative therapies. To account for the psychological and social aspects of the clinical effects, *cost-utility* analyses are designed to include quality of life measures (e.g. quality-adjusted life years). Finally, *cost-benefit* analyses are designed to compare the net costs and clinical effects, with all outcomes expressed in monetary values. It should be noted that the net cost of therapy may take into account direct future health care costs (e.g., hospitalization or other health care utilization) as well as indirect costs (e.g., loss of productivity, caregiver time) and psychological or social costs (pain, depression, anxiety). The appropriate use of indirect costs in health economic evaluations is somewhat controversial, due to the difficulty of estimating the true costs of lost productivity (Koopmanschap et al., 1993); however, these outcomes may be particularly significant in the assessment of conditions associated with long-term disability or early mortality.

Pharmacoeconomic data can be collected in a variety of research settings. One strategy is to include pharmacoeconomic outcome measures in randomized controlled trials of the investigational compound, as part of the clinical drug development program (Data et al., 1995). As health care providers may desire pharmacoeconomic information at the time of product registration, this option represents an opportunity to collect such data prior to approval. However, there are some difficulties with this approach. As randomized controlled trials are conducted under "idealized" conditions, results may not be predictive of economic outcomes in "real life." In addition, for therapies which treat chronic, life-long conditions such as diabetes, pharmacoeconomic analyses may require a very large study population and several years to determine drug effects on relevant long-term outcome measures. In patients with diabetes, for example, the highest costs are attributable to end-stage complications that may require years or decades of assessment. Thus, the assessment of such long-term variables may require the use of economic models based on intermediate end-points.

Post-approval trials provide an opportunity to collect pharmacoeconomic data in a more diverse group of patients and/or in a more naturalistic setting. These prospective studies can be conducted to confirm previous findings or to address new research questions. However, relaxed protocol restraints may result in lower internal validity than a randomized controlled trial. Finally, as use of the new drug becomes more widespread, retrospective data provide another source of pharmacoeconomic data, but only particular types of information may be accessible with this type of analysis.

Few results of pharmacoeconomic studies involving antidiabetic therapies have been published. However, interest in this area of research is clearly increasing. A cost-effectiveness analysis of intensive and conventional therapy in type 1 diabetic patients was recently completed, based on the results of the DCCT (DCCT Research Group, 1996). Because the DCCT was not long enough and was not designed to evaluate reductions in end-stage complications or mortality, a simulation model was used to project the incidence of microvascular and neurologic complications in a hypothetical sample of 10,000 individuals with type 1 diabetes. The analysis showed that while the estimated lifetime cost of intensive therapy per patient was \$33,746 greater than conventional therapy, the cost per year of life gained was \$28,661. When length of life was adjusted for quality of life, the costs of intensive therapy were \$19,987 greater than conventional therapy for each quality-adjusted life year gained. Based on guidelines that have been used to evaluate other medical treatments in the U.S., these figures were within the range of cost-effectiveness thought to represent a good value (Laupacis et al., 1992).

Another recent study assessed the health economic benefits of good glycemic control in patients with type 2 diabetes (Testa & Simonson, 1998). In this randomized, double-blind trial, 569 patients were randomized to receive diet therapy and extended-release glipizide (Glucotrol XL$^®$) or placebo for 12 weeks. In addition to evaluations of glycemic control, short-term pharmacoeconomic variables including productivity and quality of life were measured. At the end of the study, mean HbA_{1c} and fasting blood glucose levels were reduced with glipizide in comparison to placebo ($p<0.001$). Treatment differences on quality of life measures, including symptom distress ($p<0.001$), general perceived health ($p=0.004$), cognitive function ($p=0.005$), and an overall visual analog scale ($p=0.04$), also favored glipizide. Finally, glipizide resulted in significantly ($p<0.001$) higher retained employment (97% versus 85%), greater productive capacity or mean days worked per group (99% versus 87%), and lower absenteeism (losses of \$24 versus \$115 per worker per month). The costs of therapy were not evaluated in this study. Thus, although the economic benefits of anti-hyperglycemic therapy are generally associated with reductions in long-term medical expenses due to complications, the results of this study suggest that there may also be immediate economic and quality-of-life benefits associated with good glycemic control in type 2 diabetic patients.

Although not a basis for drug approval in the U.S., pharmacoeconomic information that is directly related to an approved indication may be provided to formulary committees or similar entities, if it is based on competent and reliable scientific evidence (FDA Modernization Act 1997, Section 114). However, as the field of health economic research is relatively young, there are no existing standards or guidelines for the methodology of pharmacoeconomic studies. Some challenges associated with designing pharmacoeconomic analyses include the identification of relevant costs and clinical consequences, the selection of appropriate comparator therapies, and the effective use of sensitivity analyses to test assumptions (Drummond, 1996; Lee & Sanchez, 1991). In order to optimize the utility of pharmacoeconomic studies, a consensus regarding these and other issues will need to be achieved.

References

Cutler NR, Sramek JJ, Kilborn JR. The bridging concept: optimizing the dose for phase II/III in Alzheimer's disease. *Neurodegeneration* 1996; **5**(4): 511–514.

Cutler NR, Sramek JJ, Kurtz NM, Murphy MF, Carta A. *Accelerating CNS Drug Development*. Chichester: John Wiley & Sons, 1998.

Cutler NR, Sramek JJ. Scientific and ethical concerns in clinical trials in Alzheimer's patients: the bridging study. *Eur J Clin Pharmacol* 1995; **48**: 421–428.

Cutler NR, Sramek JJ. Guidelines for conducting bridging studies in Alzheimer's disease. *Alzheimer Dis Assoc Disord* 1998; **12**(2): 88–92.

Cutler NR, Sramek JJ, Kurtz NM. *Anxiolytic Compounds: Perspectives in Drug Development.* Chichester: John Wiley & Sons, 1996.

Cutler NR, Sramek JJ, Veroff AE. *Alzheimer's Disease: Optimizing Drug Development Strategies.* Chichester: John Wiley & Sons, 1994.

Cutler NR, Sramek JJ, Greenblatt DJ, Chaikin P, Ford N, Lesko LJ, Davis B, Williams RL. Defining the maximum tolerated dose: investigator, academic, industry and regulatory perspectives. *J Clin Pharmacol* 1997; **37**: 767–783.

Data JL, Willke RJ, Barnes JR, DiRoma PJ. Re-engineering drug development: integrating pharmacoeconomic research into the drug development process. *Psychopharm Bull* 1995; **31**(1): 67–73.

DCCT Research Group. Lifetime benefits and costs of intensive therapy as practiced in the Diabetes Control and Complications Trial. *JAMA* 1996; **276**(17): 1409–1415.

Drummond MF. The future of pharmacoeconomics: bridging science and practice. *Clin Ther* 1996; **18**(5): 969–978.

Fischer S, Hanefeld M, Spengler M, Boehme K, Temelkova-Kurktschiev T. European study on dose-response relationship of acarbose as a first-line drug in non-insulin-dependent diabetes mellitus: efficacy and safety of low and high doses. *Acta Diabetol* 1998; **35**(1): 34–40.

Garber AJ, Duncan TG, Goodman AM, Mills DJ, Rohlf JL. Efficacy of metformin in type II diabetes: results of a double-blind, placebo-controlled, dose-response trial. *Am J Med* 1997; **103**(6): 491–497.

Goldberg RB, Holvey SM, Schneider J. A dose-response study of glimepiride in patients with NIDDM who have previously received sulfonylurea agents. The Glimepiride Protocol #201 Study Group. *Diabetes Care* 1996; **19**(8): 849–856.

Koopmanschap MA, Rutten FFH. The indirect costs in economic studies: confronting the confusion. *Pharmacoeconomics* 1993; **4**: 446–454.

Laupacis A, Feeny D, Detsky AS, Tugwell PX. How attractive does a new technology have to be to warrant adoption and utilization? Tentative guidelines for using clinical and economic evaluations. *CMAJ* 1992; **146**(4): 473–481.

Lee JT, Sanchez LA. Interpretation of "cost-effective" and soundness of economic evaluations in the pharmacy literature. *Am J Hosp Pharm* 1991; **48**(12): 2622–2627.

Murphy MF, Sramek JJ, Kurtz NM, Carta A, Cutler NR. *Alzheimer's Disease: Optimizing the Development of the Next Generation of Therapeutic Compounds.* London: Greenwich Medical Media Ltd., 1998.

Scott AR, Tattersall RB. Alpha-glucosidase inhibition in the treatment of non-insulin-dependent diabetes mellitus. *Diabet Med* 1988; **5**(1): 42–46.

Sramek JJ, Cutler NR, Kurtz NM, Murphy MF, Carta A. *Optimizing the Development of Antipsychotic Drugs*. Chichester: John Wiley & Sons, 1997.

Testa MA, Simonson DC. Health economic benefits and quality of life during improved glycemic control in patients with type 2 diabetes mellitus. *JAMA* 1998; **280**(17): 1490–1496.

Weissman L. Multiple-dose phase I trials–normal volunteers or patients? One viewpoint. *J Clin Pharmacol* 1981; **21**(10): 385–387.

13

CONCLUDING REMARKS

Over the past decade, therapeutic development in diabetes has taken on a new urgency. The landmark results of the Diabetes Control and Complications Trial (DCCT) and United Kingdom Prospective Diabetes Study (UKPDS) provided evidence of the link between metabolic control and diabetic complications, emphasizing the importance of anti-hyperglycemic therapies. In addition, substantial progress has been made towards the development of the first compounds designed to directly treat or prevent diabetic complications. With the rising incidence of type 1 diabetes and the projected global increase in type 2 diabetes, it is likely that the need for safe and effective antidiabetic therapies will only continue to grow into the next century.

With the significant progress that has been made into the determination of factors involved in the pathogenesis of diabetes, disease prevention has become a major focus of research for the first time. Potential risk factors have been identified that could provide the opportunity for early intervention. Several strategies are under investigation for type 1 diabetes, including the induction of immunotolerance and protection of the β-cell. For patients at risk for type 2 disease, insulin-sensitizing compounds are being tested as an additional option to diet and exercise. The prospect of preventing or slowing disease development represents an exciting new area of exploration, and will likely remain a research priority.

Therapeutic development for the treatment of type 2 diabetes has also made significant strides, with the approval of several novel drug classes and compounds. Some of these therapies (e.g. metformin, troglitazone) address the root of the disease, namely insulin resistance, and all appear to have a lower liability for the side effects associated with insulin therapy (e.g., hypoglycemia and weight gain). Although it can be argued that no current therapy is ideal, these new underlying approaches have provided the basis for the development of safer and more effective compounds.

One clear trend for the future of therapeutics in diabetes is the development of compounds to prevent or treat long-term complications. Several approaches are under clinical investigation, including anti-glycation compounds, aldose reductase inhibitors, aminoguanidines, anti-ischemics, and carnitine activators. These strategies have the potential to provide the first direct pharmaceutical treatment options for diabetic patients with microvascular complications. However, the development of these compounds will require parallel innovations in clinical trial design. As no standard surrogate endpoints have been established for the assessment of diabetic complications, some consensus will need to be achieved in order to meaningfully evaluate the clinical efficacy of these compounds.   Additionally, further exploration of neuropsychological endpoints and diabetes-related cognitive dysfunction will be necessary to more comprehensively assess treatment response in this patient population.

The recent FDA draft guidance for the evaluation of antidiabetic therapies has also highlighted several methodological issues that require further consideration.   Areas of particular significance include the use of placebo or active controls in pivotal efficacy trials, and standards for demonstrating efficacy. It is hoped that the finalization of this document will help to optimize the development process by clarifying regulatory expectations. Additionally, the use of early exploratory designs, such as the bridging study, is expected to further streamline the development of antidiabetic therapies.

Diabetes is a public health crisis with an urgent need for safer and more effective therapies. Although the treatment of diabetes has come a long way since the discovery of insulin by Banting and Best, the optimization of therapeutic strategies remains a challenge that will require the combined efforts of those in academia, industry, and the regulatory arena.

INDEX

oral insulin 53
outcome measures 132 — 4

pain assessment 144, 148 — 50
paresthesia assessment 144, 148
patient exposure for drug approval 131
peripheral polyneuropathy 27, 167
peripheral vascular disease 28
peroneal motor nerve conduction
    velocity 144 — 5, 150, 151
pharmoeconomic approaches 182 — 3
phenformin 29, 56, 89, 91, 92
    cardiovascular event risk 92, 93
photocoagulation 26
pimagedine 117
pioglitazone 57, 116 — 17
placebo controlled studies 129 — 30
ponalrestat 80
pramlintide 59, 113 — 14
preventive strategies
    type 1 diabetes 37 — 41
    type 2 diabetes 41 — 2
Profile of Mood States (POMS) 148
protein glycation 76
    microangiopathy 23
protein kinase C inactivation 23
proteinuria 26, 155
    captopril therapy 154, 155

quality of life assessment 147 — 8
quantitative autonomic testing 144
quantitative sensory testing 144

ramipril 81
Rapid Visual Information Processing
    (RVIP) 165
rapid-acting insulin analogs 50 — 1
repaglinide 58, 102 — 3, 135
residual β-cell function 38 — 9
retinopathy 23, 24 — 6
    assessment 139 — 41, 156
    glycemic control relationship 138
    grading system 24, 25
    incidence 137 — 8
    laser therapy 141 — 2, 143
    medical therapy trials 141, 142, 143
    preventive strategies 25, 47
    surgery 26
Right Hemisphere Scale 171
rosiglitazone 57, 115 — 16

rubella, congenital syndrome 5

sedentary lifestyle 9
seven-standard field fundus photography
    140, 156
Short-Form 36-item Health Survey
    (SF-36) 148
Sickness Impact Profile (SIP) 147
Sorbinil Retinopathy Study 141
Spatial Memory Scale 171
statins 29
stereo fundus photography 141
stroke 28
sulfonylureas 29, 54 — 5
    long-term safety 135
sural nerve biopsy 144
sural nerve conduction velocity 145 — 6
syndrome X 28

thiazolidinediones 57 — 8
tolbutamide 29, 134
    cardiovascular event risk 99
tolrestat 81
Total Symptom Score (TSS) 149
tricyclic antidepressants 28
TRIPOD 41 — 2
troglitazone 41 — 2, 57, 99 — 102
    safety 57 — 8, 102 — 3, 135
truncated nerve growth factor receptor
    144, 148

United Kingdom Prospective Diabetes
    Study (UKPDS) 99, 132, 134, 135,
    187
urine glucose 75

vascular endothelial growth factor
    (VEGF) 25
Verbal Memory Scale 170 — 1
viral causative factors 5
Visual Analog Scale (VAS) 149 — 50
vitrectomy 26
voglibose 111 — 13

zenarestat 117 — 18
zopolrestat 118
Zung Self-Rating Depression Scale 168